# New Perspectives on Health, Disability, Welfare and the Labour Market

*Edited by*

Colin Lindsay, Bent Greve,
Ignazio Cabras, Nick Ellison
and Stephen Kellett

**WILEY** Blackwell

This edition first published 2015
Originally published as Volume 49, Issue 2 of *Social Policy & Administration*
Book compilation © 2015 John Wiley & Sons Ltd

*Registered Office*
John Wiley & Sons Ltd, The Atrium, Southern Gate, Chichester, West Sussex, PO19 8SQ, UK

*Editorial Offices*
350 Main Street, Malden, MA 02148-5020, USA
9600 Garsington Road, Oxford, OX4 2DQ, UK
The Atrium, Southern Gate, Chichester, West Sussex, PO19 8SQ, UK

For details of our global editorial offices, for customer services, and for information about how to apply for permission to reuse the copyright material in this book please see our website at www.wiley.com/wiley-blackwell.

Library of Congress Cataloging-in-Publication data is available for this book.

ISBN 9781119145516 (paperback)

A catalogue record for this book is available from the British Library.

Cover image: Maxiphoto/Getty

Set in 10.5/11pt NewBaskervilleStd by Aptara Inc., New Delhi, India
Printed and bound in Malaysia by Vivar Printing Sdn Bhd

1    2015

# New Perspectives on Health, Disability, Welfare and the Labour Market

**Broadening Perspectives on Social Policy**
*Series Editor: Bent Greve*

The object of this series, in this age of re-thinking on social welfare, is to bring fresh points of view and to attract fresh audiences to the mainstream of social policy debate.

The choice of themes is designed to feature issues of major interest and concern, such as are already stretching the boundaries of social policy.

This is the nineteenth collection of papers in the series. Previous volumes include:

- Contracting-out Welfare Services: Comparing National Policy Designs for Unemployment Assistance *M. Considine and S. O'Sullivan*
- Evidence and Evaluation in Social Policy *I. Greener and B. Greve*
- Crime and Social Policy *H. Kemshall*
- The Times They Are Changing? Crisis and the Welfare State *B. Greve*
- Reforming Long-term Care in Europe *J. Costa-Font*
- Choice: Challenges and Perspectives for the European Welfare States *B. Greve*
- Living in Dangerous Times: Fear, Insecurity, Risk and Social Policy *D. Denney*
- Reforming the Bismarckian Welfare Systems *B. Palier and C. Martin*
- Challenging Welfare Issues in the Global Countryside *G. Giarchi*
- Migration, Immigration and Social Policy *C. Jones Finer*
- Overstretched: European Families Up Against The Demands of Work and Care *T. Kröger and J. Sipilä*
- Making a European Welfare State?: Convergences and Conflicts over European Social Policy *P. Taylor-Gooby*
- The Welfare of Food: Rights and Responsibilities in a Changing World *E. Dowler and C. Jones Finer*
- Environmental Issues and Social Welfare *M. Cahill and T. Fitzpatrick*
- The Business of Research: Issues of Policy and Practice *C. Jones Finer and G. Lewando Hundt*
- New Risks, New Welfare: Signposts for Social Policy *N. Manning and I. Shaw*
- Transnational Social Policy *C. Jones Finer*
- Crime & Social Exclusion *C. Jones Finer and M. Nellis*

# CONTENTS

Contents

# LIST OF CONTRIBUTORS

**Ben Baumberg,** School of Social Policy, Sociology & Social Research, University of Kent, Canterbury, UK

**Christina Beatty,** Centre for Regional Economic and Social Research, Sheffield Hallam University, Sheffield, UK

**Ignazio Cabras,** University of Northumbria, Newcastle, UK

**Jenny Ceolta-Smith,** School of Health Sciences, University of Salford, Salford, UK

**Mike Danson,** Department of Business Management, Heriot-Watt University, Edinburgh, UK

**Nick Ellison,** University of York, York, UK

**Steve Fothergill,** Centre for Regional Economic and Social Research, Sheffield Hallam University, Sheffield, UK

**Kayleigh Garthwaite,** Department of Geography, University of Durham, Durham, UK

**Bent Greve,** Roskilde University, Roskilde, Denmark

**Stephen Kellett,** Centre for Psychological Services Research, University of Sheffield, UK and Sheffield Health and Social Care NHS Foundation Trust, Sheffield, UK

**Colin Lindsay,** University of Strathclyde, Glasgow, UK

**Ailsa McKay,** Glasgow School for Business and Society, Glasgow Caledonian University, Glasgow, UK

**Fiona Purdie,** Department of Clinical Psychology, University of Leeds, Leeds, UK and Psychology Services, Bradford Teaching Hospitals NHS Foundation Trust, Bradford, UK

**Sarah Salway,** School of Health and Related Research, Sheffield Hallam University, Sheffield, UK

**Willie Sullivan,** Common Weal, Biggar, UK

**Matt Sutton,** Manchester Centre for Health Economics, University of Manchester, Manchester, UK

**Angela Mary Tod,** Faculty of Medical and Human Sciences, University of Manchester, Manchester, UK

**William Whittaker,** Manchester Centre for Health Economics, University of Manchester, Manchester, UK

# Introduction:
## New Perspectives on Health, Disability, Welfare and the Labour Market

**Colin Lindsay, Bent Greve, Ignazio Cabras,
Nick Ellison and Stephen Kellett**

## Introduction

More than 2.4 million people of working age in the UK are out of work and claiming 'incapacity' or disability benefits (DBs). Reducing the high levels of benefit claiming among those with health limitations and disabilities has been a priority for successive governments (Lindsay and Houston 2013). Other countries of the Organisation for Economic Co-operation and Development (OECD), ranging from Sweden, with its 'social democratic' welfare state (Hagelund and Bryngelson 2014), to the 'liberal' USA also report high rates of disability claiming, and have similarly prioritized measures to bring down welfare rolls (Milligan 2012). Given this context, policy debates have focused on both reforms to the administration of DBs and the content of targeted activation (Bannink 2014).

Recent policy responses in the UK have taken the form of measures to restrict access to welfare benefits and impose increased compulsory 'work-related activity' on claimants. However, current policy arguably fails to reflect the evidence that people on long-term DBs face a complex combination of barriers to work and social inclusion. The evidence points to a multi-dimensional form of disadvantage, requiring a holistic, joined-up policy response – claimants may struggle to manage a range of disabilities and health conditions (with mental health problems widespread); many report gaps in employability and skills; and, *crucially*, claiming is spatially concentrated in communities characterized by poor health and labour markets that have fewer (and fewer high quality) job

*New Perspectives on Health, Disability, Welfare and the Labour Market*, First Edition.
Edited by Colin Lindsay, Bent Greve, Ignazio Cabras, Nick Ellison and Stephen Kellett.
© 2015 John Wiley & Sons, Ltd. Published 2015 by John Wiley & Sons, Ltd.

opportunities. Many of these challenges are present in other European and OECD welfare states, where there are similar tensions between activation policies that seek to drive sick and disabled people off benefits and into work, and the challenges faced by these people to manage conditions and sustain their position in the labour market.

There is a need for continuing inter-disciplinary research on the nature of the 'disability benefits problem' and the efficacy of current policy solutions and public services. This Special Issue brings together researchers who seek to explore the distinctive, yet interrelated, elements of the problems faced by disability claimants, and evaluate related policies and services. The Special Issue is co-edited by an inter-disciplinary team drawn from the fields of social policy, economics, sociology and clinical psychology. A seminar series supported by the White Rose University Consortium allowed many of the authors to share early versions of their articles.

## Content of the Special Issue

All of articles that follow connect with key issues around the complex combination of health, employability, workplace and labour market-related factors that explain DB claiming in disadvantaged areas and among vulnerable groups. The Special Issue opens with a review of evidence conducted by the co-editors. We present the most up-to-date and robust evidence on the nature of the DB problem in the UK. While drawing upon frameworks presented by previous studies (Beatty *et al.* 2009; Lindsay and Houston 2011, 2013), we also identify important new and emerging evidence, for example in relation to the impact of poor quality jobs on working-age health, and how labour market casualization has contributed to DB claiming. The other contribution of this first article is a comparative analysis of the disability activation and welfare reform agenda in a very different welfare state – Denmark. Here, we acknowledge that, despite a greater readiness to intervene in the workplace (through initiatives such as the flex-jobs programme), policymakers have similarly struggled to arrive at solutions that address the disadvantage faced by disabled people. We conclude that more radical solutions may be required to deliver genuine equality of opportunity in the mainstream labour market, and to stimulate sufficient labour demand in regions and welfare states where there are simply too few decent jobs.

The next three articles in this Special Issue analyze aspects of the 'DB problem' from a range of theoretical and disciplinary starting points. Christina Beatty and Steve Fothergill take a long-view of the rise in disability claimant numbers in the UK since the 1970s, and conclude that spatial concentrations of health and disability-related worklessness have proved largely impervious to successive waves of welfare reform. However, they also note that increased conditionality in access to benefits (the centrepiece of the current UK policy agenda) risks driving the most vulnerable out of the system, resulting in increased social risk. Only policies designed to address ill-health and disability, combined with demand-side labour market interventions, can help to empower DB claimants to progress towards meaningful work.

Ben Baumberg presents in-depth, qualitative data to demonstrate how lower skilled workers in disadvantaged labour markets are less able to access the kind of workplace adjustments that might otherwise allow them to cope with health or disability-related limitations. Baumberg's research thus reiterates the multi-dimensional character of the potential barriers faced by DB claimants, which are rooted not only in health limitations and disability, but also structural labour market and workplace factors. Kayleigh Garthwaite also draws on qualitative research, exploring experiences of poverty, social isolation and stigma among the DB claimant group – a grim reality at odds with the popular mythology of a feckless underclass choosing life on benefits. Will Whittaker and Matt Sutton provide further quantitative evidence demonstrating that the health limitations of DB claimants are *real*. Whittaker's and Sutton's longitudinal analysis of British Household Panel Survey data highlights the particular importance of mental ill-health in explaining high rates of DB claiming over time.

The final three articles return to a more explicit focus on evaluating and informing current policy. First, Fiona Purdie and Stephen Kellett present the results of extensive survey research with DB claimants participating in condition management programmes designed and delivered by health professionals. They identify well-being and employability benefits for many of those participating, reinforcing the message that health-related support should be central to policies to address the DB problem. Purdie and Kellett also, however, acknowledge differences in the outcomes achieved for sub-groups among those on DBs, arguing for further research to inform a broader range of health services targeting people on working-age benefits. Within the UK policy context, we appear to be some way off the establishment of such holistic and broad-based health interventions. Indeed, the article by Jenny Ceolta-Smith, Sarah Salway and Angela Mary Tod on the Work Programme in the UK suggests that access to health-related support is likely to be partial and unequal among the DB claimant group. Lastly, the article by Mike Danson, Ailsa McKay and Willie Sullivan offers a macro-level, comparative perspective on worklessness and inequality. This final article identifies lessons from some of Europe's more equal societies and argues for a fundamental recalibration of welfare and economic policies in the UK to address entrenched inequalities. It is an eloquent and impassioned argument reflecting the commitment to policies for a fairer society that defined the career of our late and greatly respected colleague (and article co-author) Professor Ailsa McKay.

The UK, like many other welfare states, faces a continuing problem of high levels of disability claiming. In the longer term, policymakers will also be required to respond to the challenge of helping an ageing labour force to work for longer, which will inevitably mean managing health conditions and disabilities in the workplace. Current policy in the UK focuses almost entirely on restricting access to benefits and imposing work-first activation in order to address imagined behavioural deficits among claimants. These policies may achieve the short-term goal of driving some vulnerable people out of the welfare system, but there is little evidence that they can provide routes into sustainable employment. A new policy agenda is required, which addresses the complex combination of health, employability, workplace and labour market-related factors that explain the UK's DB problem. Our duty as social policy researchers is to marshal the evidence from across disciplines in the hope of informing appropriate policies. This Special Issue seeks to make a small contribution to that shared goal.

## References

Bannink, D. (2014), Social policy from Olson to Ostrom: a case study of Dutch disability insurance, *Social Policy & Administration*, 48, 3: 279–99.

Beatty, C., Fothergill, S., Houston, D., Powell, R. and Sissons, P. (2009), A gendered theory of employment, unemployment and sickness, *Environment and Planning C: Government and Policy*, 27, 6: 958–74.

Hagelund, A. and Bryngelson, A. (2014), Change and resilience in welfare state policy: the politics of sickness insurance in Norway and Sweden, *Social Policy & Administration*, 48, 3: 300–18.

Lindsay, C. and Houston, D. (2011), Fit for purpose? Welfare reform and challenges for health and labour market policy in the UK, *Environment and Planning A*, 43, 3:703–21.

Lindsay, C. and Houston, D. (2013), *Disability Benefits, Welfare Reform and Employment Policy*, Basingstoke: Palgrave Macmillan.

Milligan, K. (2012), The long-run growth of disability insurance in the United States. In D. Wise (ed.), *Social Security Programs and Retirement Around the World*, Chicago, IL: University of Chicago Press, pp. 359–89.

# 1

# Assessing the Evidence Base on Health, Employability and the Labour Market – Lessons for Activation in the UK

## Colin Lindsay, Bent Greve, Ignazio Cabras, Nick Ellison and Stephen Kellett

## Introduction

Despite recent attempts by UK policymakers to restrict access to incapacity and disability benefits (DBs),[1] claimant numbers remain high by historical comparison, with approximately 2.4 million people receiving these forms of income support in 2014. The need for policy action to assist people on DBs is not disputed. Spending long periods on these benefits has been associated with further deteriorations in health (Bambra 2011); the meagreness of payment rates in countries such as the UK means that claimants experience increased poverty risks (Kemp and Davidson 2010); and exclusion from work may undermine individuals' employability (Green and Shuttleworth 2013). However, there remain concerns that current policy agendas are not equal to the task of moving large numbers of people from DBs into sustainable employment. Indeed, the main focus of UK Government policy appears to be on restricting access to DBs by tightening eligibility criteria and means-testing. There appears little sign of a coherent strategy to enhance the employability and health of those already on benefits (other than directing claimants to a generic, compulsory activation programme – The Work Programme – or other forms of 'work-related activity') (Lindsay and Houston 2013).

This article aims to offer direction on more productive foci for welfare reform and activation policies. We do this by reviewing the latest evidence on the 'nature of the problem' (i.e. the factors contributing to high levels of DBs among some groups and communities); analyzing

*New Perspectives on Health, Disability, Welfare and the Labour Market*, First Edition.
Edited by Colin Lindsay, Bent Greve, Ignazio Cabras, Nick Ellison and Stephen Kellett.
© 2015 John Wiley & Sons, Ltd. Published 2015 by John Wiley & Sons, Ltd.

the appropriateness of current and recent policies in responding to these factors; and (briefly) contrasting the UK's approach with that of Denmark, which has deployed a different set of policy instruments in its efforts to reduce DB numbers. In order to conduct this analysis of the nature of the problem and evaluation of policy solutions, we carried out a structured literature and evidence review identifying the most robust evidence from both academic sources and policy stakeholders. We used online search engines to identify key research and policy publications with keywords including 'activation', 'active labour market programme', 'incapacity benefits', 'disability benefits', 'welfare-to-work', and variants on these themes. Following a preliminary thematic review of outputs, we selected out key research reports and academic publications to provide the focus for our analysis because of their specific interest in the challenges, outcomes, benefits, limitations and lessons from employability programmes targeting those on DBs. The reliability of this approach was strengthened by its coverage of research from a range of disciplines (reflecting the multi-disciplinary expertise of the authors) including economic geography, social policy, clinical psychology and public health policy analysis. Our findings are presented below. The analysis also draws on the latest research published in this Special Issue of *Social Policy & Administration*. The article then concludes with a discussion of implications for future policy development.

## Assessing the Evidence Base: Factors behind Concentrations of Disability Claiming

Over the past decade, successive UK Governments have deployed *relatively* consistent policies to address high levels of DB claiming. The focus of policy has been on restricting access to, and increasing the conditionality associated with, welfare benefits, along with a greater emphasis on activation, first under the Pathways to Work (PtW) initiative (2003–10) and now the Work Programme, the main activation programme for people of working age. However, it has been suggested that the general thrust of policy fails to address the complex combination of factors that explain concentrations of dB claiming (Beatty *et al.* 2009). Following Lindsay's and Houston's (2013) line of argument, we now assess the latest evidence on the extent to which three key issues can be identified as underlying the high level of DBs claiming in the UK, namely: concentrations of health and disability-related barriers among the claimant group; gaps in their employability and skills; and labour market inequalities and the impact of low quality work on opportunities for people with health and disability-related limitations. We then go on to discuss the failure of policymakers to develop joined-up, spatially-focused solutions to these problems.

### Health and disability-related barriers

One of the distinctive features of the discourse around DBs in the UK is policymakers' reluctance to fully acknowledge that those claiming

these benefits are, indeed, sick or disabled. Policymakers partly justified this position with reference to a well-established evidence base
suggesting that industrial restructuring and job destruction in regions
dependent on traditional employment sectors preceded increases in DB
claiming. Seminal works during the mid-1990s by Beatty and Fothergill
(1994) and Green (1994) identified concentrations of DB growth in
post-industrial labour markets, suggesting that Incapacity Benefit (IB,
then the main DB) was absorbing displaced workers and hiding the
real level of unemployment. These authors wished to expose the 'hidden unemployment' problem in order to demonstrate the need for
regional demand-side policies to generate more job opportunities for
those trapped on benefits (Beatty *et al.* 2000), but their argument has
been appropriated by the political right as evidence of malingering
(CSJ 2009).

Yet this is a misrepresentation of both the evidence and the argument. Indeed, Beatty *et al.*'s (2000, 2009) seminal 'theory of employment, unemployment and sickness' hypothesized that 'hidden sickness'
was as important as 'hidden unemployment' in explaining high disability claiming in some regions. They argued that there is substantial ill-
health and work-limiting disability throughout the labour force – among
those in work, jobseekers who are available for work, and those receiving DBs. Labour market conditions decide whether those with health
or disability-related barriers are able to find their way into work (due to
employers' willingness to adjust their demands in tight labour markets)
and manage their conditions in the workplace. But this need not lead
us to conclude those on DBs are feigning illness.

Rather, there is substantial evidence as to the reality of the health and
disability-related problems faced by people claiming DBs. Ill-health or
limiting disability is consistently found as the primary reason why most
DB claimants exit work in the first place, with extant health conditions
then also a key barrier to return to work (Beatty *et al.* 2010; Kemp and
Davidson 2010). Claimants with multiple and/or more serious conditions are significantly more likely to be 'permanently sick' (i.e. remain
on benefits), in contrast to those with fewer conditions who are more
likely to find work (Barnes and Sissons 2013). For those re-entering
employment following a period on DB, but then failing to sustain work,
a decline in health is a common feature (Dixon and Warrener 2008).
Large-scale national population surveys such as the British Household
Panel Survey (BHPS) suggest robust and long-term relationships
between health and exclusion from work (Jones *et al.* 2010), although
as noted elsewhere in this Special Issue these data also highlight
the importance of interactions between ill-health and spatial labour
demand inequalities (Whittaker and Sutton 2015). Robroek *et al.*'s
(2013) analysis of older workers' trajectories in 11 countries based on
the 'Survey of Health, Ageing, and Retirement in Europe' confirms that
poor health and health behaviours as well as other work-related factors
may all play a role in exits from paid employment, although their
significance may vary according to exit routes. There is a significant

relationship between DB claiming and physical (Bambra 2011) and psychiatric mortality (McKee-Ryan *et al.* 2005).

National Health Service (NHS) professionals working with DB claimants confirm evidence of a broad range of interacting and comorbid health problems and disabilities (Lindsay and Dutton 2013). Other researchers have similarly used accepted clinical tools (such as the 'Hospital Anxiety and Depression Scale') to identify significantly poorer health among the DB claimant population that appears resistant to increasing exposure to conditionality and/or 'incentives' as part of changes to the benefits system (Garthwaite *et al.* 2014). Purdie and Kellett (2015) evidence the pre-treatment severity of health problems and also register rates of associated clinically significant improvements following interventions to enable claimants to better manage their conditions. However, Rick *et al.* (2008) note that there are few well supported conclusions that can be made concerning the efficacy of health interventions to help DB recipients return to work, because the extant studies lacked credible outcome methodologies. Therefore, more methodologically robust outcome studies of health interventions with distressed claimants need to be conducted, in order to enable further meta-analytic perspectives to be taken. In summary, there is powerful evidence that health and disability-related limitations reported by those on DBs are real and an ongoing aspect of life without work. As we confirm below, other factors – and crucially the nature and extent of labour demand – tend to define whether such health and disability-related barriers can be managed in the workplace, or alternatively exclude people from the world of work.

### Employability-related barriers

We see above that, contrary to some policymakers' claims, health and disability-related barriers are key to understanding the nature of the DB problem. Yet, successive UK Governments have been keener to portray the problem as rooted in the attitudes and behaviour of claimants. As we see below, increased conditionality and compulsion in the DB system appear to reflect a consensus among policymakers on the need to use financial incentives and punitive sanctions 'to generate positive behavioural effects' (DWP 2010: 10). From a behavioural theory point of view, policymakers rely heavily (or exclusively) on punishment, as opposed to reward contingencies, as a means of changing the work behaviours of DB claimants.

The evidence for the existence of a 'dependency culture' among DB claimants is, however, limited. Beatty *et al.*'s (2010) extensive survey research with DB claimants deployed a raft of attitudinal questions to assess work beliefs and found little evidence for negative or low levels of work commitment. Nor were DB claimants expert in 'playing the system (i.e. particularly knowledgeable about benefit regulations). Such findings enhance a long-established evidence base contradicting the rhetoric of individual claimants 'choosing to live on benefits' and popular myths of families defined and populated by multiple generations of the unemployed (Shildrick *et al.* 2012). Rather, evidence from in-depth research with DB claimants finds recurring themes of poverty and insecurity whilst struggling financially to survive on benefits, with experiences of the benefits system (and especially increasing conditionality) defined by stigma and distress (Garthwaite *et al.* 2014).

That said, people on DBs tend to hold a variety of views about work. Green and Shuttleworth (2013) found that a range of factors (most notably age and health) shape claimants' optimism and level of commitment to work. Kemp's and Davidson's (2010) longitudinal research similarly identified differences in levels of work commitment amongst the DB group, although other variables related to health and employability were much more powerful predictors of individuals' chances of returning to the labour market. Webster *et al.* (2013) argue that perceptions of the severity of limitations imposed by health conditions and the state of the local labour market can interact to produce pessimistic self-evaluations of both health and employability.

So attitudes to work vary considerably – but there is limited evidence that individual motivation or commitment are decisive in explaining the significant labour market exclusion experienced by those on DBs. Nevertheless, there is stronger evidence that long-term DB claimants face a complex range of other employability-related barriers to work. Extensive survey work with those on DBs demonstrates that they are significantly more likely to report basic skills problems, low levels of qualification, gaps in work experience, repeated periods of unemployment and limited social network ties to those in work (Beatty *et al.* 2010, 2013; Green and Shuttleworth 2013; Kemp and Davidson 2010; Barnes and Sissons 2013). Garthwaite's (2015) research in this Special Issue provides compelling additional evidence of experiences of social isolation and poverty among DB claimants.

Such toxic combinations of employability-related barriers are common among people excluded from the labour market for long periods, and call for holistic activation programmes that are flexible in addressing the complex problems faced by disadvantaged groups. Indeed, the manner in which people on DBs often report multiple barriers and find themselves at the back of the queue for jobs means that supply-side activation is justified (Beatty and Fothergill 2015) – we simply dispute the appropriateness and capacity of current policy content to address the complex needs of many DB claimants.

*Labour market barriers*

Successive UK governments have been reluctant to acknowledge the spatial labour market inequalities that clearly shape the nature of the DB problem (Lindsay and Houston 2013). Yet, the evidence suggests that labour market inequalities are fundamental to explaining why people in certain communities are more likely to find themselves trapped on DBs. Beatty *et al.* (2000, 2009, 2010, 2013) have amassed a compelling evidence base demonstrating that DB claiming is concentrated in those regional labour markets that experienced large-scale job destruction following industrial restructuring. In post-industrial cities, the processes of job destruction associated with the decline of manufacturing were never fully reversed during the 'long boom' of the 1990s and 2000s, which produced uneven growth, often in casualized and low-paid service work (Webster *et al.* 2013). In mapping DB claiming both before and after the Employment Support Allowance (ESA) reform in the UK, Lindsay and Houston (2011: 707) similarly conclude that 'the map of claim rates corresponds to areas of former industrial decline'. There is nothing particularly distinctive about DB claimants in post-industrial labour markets, there are just many more of them (Webster *et al.* 2013). This is explained by the lack of jobs to absorb people who otherwise might be able to cope with their health conditions in the workplace. In times of 'full employment', employers adapt their expectations so that people with health and disability-related limitations are more likely to find work (Beatty *et al.* 2013).

Employers and jobs may be of broader importance in understanding the DB problem. First, employers' willingness to make necessary and/or indicated adjustments to acknowledge health limitations – such as altering job content or work environment, or allowing changes to working hours or phased returns to work – can be crucial in facilitating re-integration for people on DBs (Kemp and Davidson 2010). Claimants regularly cite the identification of a 'sympathetic employer' as central in return to work planning (Green and Shuttleworth 2010: 234). However, lower-skilled workers in poor quality jobs in particular may struggle to negotiate adjustments with their employers (Baumberg 2015), with some employers, instead, seeming more likely to target those with health limitations for redundancy (Easterlow and Smith 2003). Increasingly aggressive absence management policies may also exacerbate health conditions among existing employees, while militating against a culture of adjustment and inclusiveness that might assist those returning to work (Taylor *et al.* 2010).

The nature and quality of jobs may also negatively impact opportunities open to people with health and disability-related limitations. As noted above, post-industrial labour markets may not have enough jobs to absorb people with health problems who could, nevertheless, manage some work. Low quality jobs in these labour markets may also contribute to the DB problem and throw up barriers to work for claimants. For example, DB claiming is more likely in labour markets dominated by casualized and short-term employment, where employers can more easily 'manage out' employees with health problems (Beatty *et al.* 2009). More specifically, under-employment (where employees are unable to secure sufficient hours or pay) may feed into the DB problem. Low-paid, part-time employees whose wages fail to meet the minimum National Insurance threshold are ineligible for employer-paid Statutory Sick Pay and are therefore more vulnerable to exit work in order to claim DBs. For people at the bottom of a polarized labour market, the benefits system is therefore 'working as a functional equivalent of sick pay (Kemp and Davidson 2009: 598).

The nature of the working life in poor quality jobs is also relevant. Claims that low-paid, entry level positions remain a stepping stone to better jobs appear contradicted by 'cycling' between work and repeated benefit claiming (Barnes and Sissons 2013). Meanwhile, in workplaces that are intensified and 'lean' or where employees have little control over the standard operating procedures that define how and where they work, there may be less scope to effectively manage health conditions and stay in work (Carter *et al.* 2013). For example, work governed by 'zero hours' contracts offers little structure around which necessary health behaviours could be planned and enacted. Baumberg's (2014) research – modelling a combination of health variables drawn from the BHPS and job content data from skills surveys – presents compelling evidence that a decreasing sense of control among employees over the past two decades has contributed to ill-health and potentially higher levels of disability claiming. There are few spatial studies quantifying the impact of changing quality across different regional economies, but we might therefore hypothesize that the dominance of low quality jobs in post-industrial labour markets (Shildrick *et al.* 2012) could be an additional factor contributing to concentrations of DB.

As Patrick (2012: 313) concludes, sick and disabled people seeking to return to work 'face a range of demand-side barriers, including the impact of stigma and discrimination, physical challenges around access and transport, and issues around the availability of suitably flexible job opportunities'. Our review of evidence above adds substantially to the evidence on this final point, demonstrating that the labour market inequalities – reflected in spatial differences in both the quantity and quality of jobs – may be crucial in shaping individuals' capacity to cope with health problems or disability in the workplace.

In summary, the most recent literature, including research presented elsewhere in this Special Issue, adds to the evidence that a complex combination of factors have combined to produce concentrations of DB claiming in disadvantaged labour markets and communities. Some of these factors reflect individual barriers, but there is little evidence that these can be simplified into a dependency culture that can be addressed through punitive welfare reforms or behavioural interventions. Rather, a combination of health/disability limitations and employability-related barriers to work combine to leave some people at the back of the queue for jobs. This disadvantage is exacerbated in post-industrial labour markets where there are not enough opportunities, and where the jobs that are available represent a difficult context within which to manage conditions (and in some cases may contribute to ill-health). A coherent strategy to provide routes into sustainable employment for people on DBs will therefore require: a range of employability-related services; integrated condition management provision to assist claimants to cope with health and disability-related limitations; and spatially-focused economic development and workplace strategies designed to ensure that there are viable job opportunities for those leaving welfare to enter work. As we see below, the current UK policy agenda falls well short of meeting these demands.

### Assessing the Policy Agenda: Welfare-to-Work for People on Disability Benefits in the UK and Lessons from Abroad

*Current policy in the UK*

To what extent is the evidence presented above reflected in the UK policy agenda on helping people from DBs into work? The current policy agenda demonstrates clear continuity with work-first approaches to activation. Within such approaches, the nature of the problem is seen as mainly rooted in the individual's attitudes and behaviour, with the logical conclusion that strengthening conditionality and compulsory activation can effect positive change in and for the individual (Lindsay and Dutton 2013). The replacement of IB with ESA as the main DB for new claimants from 2008 reflected these priorities. The ESA reform restricted access to the most generous benefit replacement rates to only those assessed as facing severe health/disability barriers, who are placed into a 'Support Group'. Those assessed as less disadvantaged are placed into a 'Work-related Activity Group' where receipt of ESA is conditional on engaging in work-focused interviews and other activation provision (see discussion below). Unlike its predecessor IB, ESA's contribution-based benefit is limited to one year for the Work-related Activity Group. Those still claiming ESA after this duration are required to transfer to a means-tested version of the benefit (meaning that those with other sources of household income may be denied payment).

Central to the ESA reform was the establishment of a stricter medical assessment – the Work Capability Assessment (WCA) – as a means of determining benefit entitlement. The WCA was introduced for all new ESA claimants by the Labour Government. The Conservative-led coalition Government then committed to re-assessing all existing benefit recipients from 2011; and there is also the expectation that all ESA claimants will be repeatedly re-assessed within two years (previously, IB claimants often reported several years between benefit eligibility assessments) (Harris and Rahilly 2011). As noted above, the WCA has been designed to separate the most disadvantaged, who are directed to the Support Group and receive DBs without condition, from those who might be able to make progress towards employment and are subject to compulsory activation – the Work-related Activity Group. The measures of work capacity deployed in the WCA process explicitly sought to 'raise the bar' in order to restrict access to benefits (for a detailed discussion of WCA content and scoring, see Harris and Rahilly 2011). Government clearly communicated that its expectation was that only a small minority of claimants should be directed towards the unconditional Support Group, and in its first year of operation the WCA found only 10 per cent of claimants to be so sick or disabled as to justify this status; 24 per cent of claimants were directed to the Work-related Activity Group; and 66 per cent were judged fit for work and denied ESA.

Initial independent reviews confirmed the inadequacy of the WCA process, which was assessed as 'mechanistic', 'lacking empathy' and impractical in capturing the impacts of many chronic and/or mental health conditions (Harrington 2010: 31). These processes created the paradoxical risk of the stress of WCA creating mental health problems (and associated costs elsewhere in the health economy) or that DB claimants would become more resistant to health interventions for fear that responsivity would be taken as a prompt by WCA assessors to change their benefit status. Many claimants have been able to reverse WCA decisions on appeal (Patrick 2012), and more recent data suggests that the WCA is being applied more sensitively, probably in response to the high numbers of successful appeals.

The second, inter-connected element of the current UK model involves extending the reach of compulsory activation to many of those on DBs. The first major activation programme targeting disability claimants was PtW, piloted by the Labour Government from 2003 and rolled out fully by 2008. The initiative was initially led by Jobcentre Plus, with health-oriented condition management services organized by partner NHS organizations. As PtW was rolled out nationally, leadership of the initiative was contracted out to (mainly private sector) 'Lead Providers' in most regions, which saw the condition management component quickly marginalized within programme content (Lindsay and Dutton 2013). The main content of PtW instead centred on five compulsory work-focused interviews; and a range of voluntary work preparation programmes based on existing 'work-first' activation provision. Attendance at work-focused interviews was enforced via the threat of benefit sanctions. Condition management provision was more fragmented in those areas where PtW was led by contracted providers, which were not required to work with NHS organizations to develop health-focused interventions (Grant 2013). Overall, the national outcomes delivered by PtW were disappointing, with no significant employment effect associated with claimants' participation (NAO 2010). However, where regions had effectively integrated Department for Work and Pensions (DWP) and NHS provision to support return to work for DB claimants, the health and employment outcomes were significant (Kellett *et al.* 2011; Purdie and Kellett 2015).

From 2011, PtW and all other UK Government activation programmes were amalgamated within the Work Programme, led by multiple 'Prime Contractors'. A 'black box' funding model affords Prime Contractors considerable autonomy in shaping services, although a payment-by-results regime that offers limited up-front funding means that there is an incentive to target 'quick wins' through work-first interventions (such as short, relatively inexpensive motivational and job search courses). Accordingly, there is substantial evidence of 'creaming and parking' among Work Programme activation providers charged with improving the employability of those on DBs (HoC 2013). The meagre health-focused provision supported under PtW appears to have been further marginalized, with few Work Programme providers prioritizing condition management. At the strategic level, there is limited evidence of engagement between the DWP and the Department of Health (Ceolta-Smith *et al.* 2015). The severity of the barriers faced by many claimants, the inadequate and inappropriate funding model for the Work Programme, and the resulting 'parking' of those with health/disability-related limitations, help to explain the disappointing job outcome figures achieved by the programme for people on ESA (Rees *et al.* 2014).

It is important to note that compulsion and conditionality remain crucial components of the Work Programme's interaction with the sick and disabled (and also defines other work-related activities that can be demanded of ESA claimants). Failure to engage in work-related activity required by Work Programme providers can result in a loss of benefits for four weeks for a first offence, rising to 13 weeks for repeated non-compliance (HoC 2013). However, there is evidence that advisers working for both Jobcentre Plus and Work Programme providers have been reluctant to report 'misbehaviour' that would result in sanctions – these street-level professionals appear to be aware of both the vulnerability of many DB claimants, and that sanctioning is likely to undermine attempts to build a relationship of trust between claimant and adviser. Consequently, under both the Work Programme and its predecessor PtW, sanction rates have been relatively low (Grant 2013).

In summary, a narrow work-first focus defines current activation strategies for people on DBs. Policymakers remain reluctant to programme health provision as a central element of their approach, despite evidence as to the substantial health and disability-related limitations faced by claimants. Nor is there evidence of government interest in the role of employers – or the broader labour demand – in shaping the DB problem. It is perhaps unsurprising then that the outcomes produced by the UK Government's focus on conditionality and activation have been disappointing. As noted above, while increasing the conditions required both to access and receive benefits may reduce on-flow, there will be little progress in terms of improving people's employability or health. Yet we know from the review of evidence above, and analyses of the characteristics of returners-to-work, that improving employability and health are both key to positive transitions for DB claimants, and that labour market and workplace factors define the opportunities available to them (Barnes and Sissons 2013). We now turn to evidence from a very different welfare state – Denmark – in an attempt to identify any additional lessons that can be learned from its policy and practice in seeking to assist the sick and disabled from welfare to work.

*Lessons from abroad: current policy in Denmark*

There are a number of reasons why Denmark represents a particularly interesting counterpoint to the UK's experience. Like the UK, Denmark is often seen as in the vanguard of 'activating' European welfare states. Denmark has also grappled with high levels of DB claiming in recent years. Yet, the Danish context is clearly distinctive from the UK in some respects. Denmark's social-democratic welfare traditions are reflected in benefits that generally deliver substantially higher replacement rates than are enjoyed by disability claimants in the UK. Denmark's spending on active measures (as a percentage of gross domestic product) is the highest in the Organisation for Economic Co-operation and Development; the UK's is in the bottom third, and the lowest of any major EU economy (OECD 2013). Furthermore, while Denmark has seen some moves towards marketization in activation (Lindsay and McQuaid 2009), there is not the same private sector dominance of service delivery, and local institutions continue to facilitate a role for social partner representatives in the policy process.

As noted above, Denmark's DB claim rate has been, and remains, relatively high, with increasing reporting of mental health problems contributing to consistently large numbers claiming (OECD 2011). The Danish policy agenda has been quite different from that pursued in the UK, although large-scale positive outcomes have similarly proved elusive. Recent policies have sought to raise awareness among disability claimants of the numerous instruments available to support labour market integration (Kjeldsen *et al.* 2013). But while there are signs that recent initiatives have successfully extended the reach of activation, for example to people with mental health problems, transitions into the mainstream labour market have proved difficult to achieve. There has been a decline in the number of people on DBs since 2011, with changes to the benefit system since 2013 further restricting access and therefore on-flow. These changes have meant that those below the age of 40 cannot claim the main 'permanent' DB (except for the most severely disabled with no prospect of developing their capacity for paid work). Most claimants under 40 are, instead, required to participate in so-called 'ressourceforløb' activation activities (as are those over 40 who have not previously undertaken such activities, in order to be eligible for DBs). During participation in ressourceforløb, benefits are paid at the level of social assistance, so for younger claimants payment rates may be relatively low, and below the rate of unemployment benefit. In principle, ressourceforløb is intended to offer integrated support coordinated across the employment, education, social work and health sectors, with interventions lasting from one to five years. The Danish Government has also pointed to substantial investments in rehabilitation provision targeting the under-40s (Brix Pedersen 2013). However, take-up of ressourceforløb has been relatively low, suggesting that the promise of coordinated, holistic services has proved difficult to deliver for local authorities, which are responsible for the implementation of these and other working age activation services. There also remain concerns that the rehabilitation plans offered to younger claimants have not been fully resourced, increasing the risk of economic insecurity faced by young people with disabilities, while intensifying the pressure upon

15

them to engage in activity that may be inappropriate and beyond their capabilities.

A second distinctive strand of active measures for people with health and disability-related limitations is the 'flex-job' programme, which provides a substantial employer subsidy for workplaces supporting those with disabilities to stay in work (and which initially offered individual participants the equivalent of a full-time wage despite working reduced hours in most cases) (Etherington and Ingold 2012). Changes introduced in 2012 reduced the work-related income received by participants, which now reflects the hours of work actually performed, with a further supplementary benefit paid at a level close to the unemployment benefit level provided to top up income. While this change has the potential to expand the reach of flex-jobs for people working fewer hours, the income received by many participants will be reduced. These changes reflect concerns among policymakers as to the affordability of the flex-jobs programme, which saw a rapid expansion in take-up during the 2000s. More generally, while there are clearly attractive features associated with a flex-jobs programme that prioritizes helping people to manage conditions *in the workplace* (and which supports employers to make adjustments), there remain concerns that its subsidy element is seen as an 'easy option', detracting from efforts to place sick and disabled people in the unsubsidized, mainstream labour market (Etherington and Ingold 2012).

A range of more recent strategies have seen an emphasis on work-first activation, partly facilitated by the transfer of responsibility for the delivery of much of the employability policy agenda to local government. The result has been a:

> wave of management and governance reforms designed to advance a work-first agenda ... [including] New Public Management reforms at the municipal level, using financial incentives and performance management to encourage implementation practices emphasizing a stronger work-first approach (Larsen 2013: 109)

In common with the UK, there is also a reluctance among policymakers to acknowledge the importance of demand-side labour market factors in shaping DB claiming, perhaps suggesting that there are 'growing similarities in the policy discourses around activation' in Denmark and the UK (Etherington and Ingold 2012: 31).

Accordingly, despite successive governments' rhetoric around providing holistic and client-centred support for people on DBs, the take-up of services such as ressourceforløb has been low, while eligibility conditions and generosity of benefits are now less favourable for (especially younger) disability claimants. Similarly, the flex-jobs programme seems to reflect the need for workplace-rooted approaches to condition management identified in our discussion of the UK problem above, but also highlights the limitations of initiatives that rely too heavily on wage subsidization to create parallel labour market conditions for people with health and disability-related limitations. Danish policymakers' declared ambition to increase participation rates among the disabled has not been realized – indeed, since 2010 there has been a drop in labour market participation, especially among those with more significant disabilities (Kjeldsen *et al.* 2013). In common with other countries, including the UK, participation rates seem more responsive to labour demand fluctuations than to any specific policy targeting people with health and disability-related limitations (Grammenos 2011).

## Discussion and Conclusions

Our review above confirms a disconnect between the evidence on the nature of the DBs 'problem' and an increasingly narrow and behaviourist policy agenda implemented under successive UK governments. Policymakers have presented high numbers of people on DB as a problem of attitude and behaviours, leading to the logical conclusion of increasing conditionality in the benefits system and compulsory activation. Our review of the evidence points to a different and much messier reality. People trapped on DBs for long periods often face substantial health problems and disability-related limitations, which explain why they left the workplace, shape attitudes towards work, and influence trajectories in and out of the labour market. Many of the same people also report employability-related barriers, ranging from gaps in basic skills to isolation from vital social networks. And crucially, the geography of labour markets defines the opportunities open to DB claimants facing a combination of health and employability-related barriers. This disadvantage is accentuated in any post-industrial local labour market where jobs are characterized by casualization, insecurity, low-pay and work intensification.

The preceding literature and evidence review can be seen as largely confirmatory, adding to the analyses presented in previous multi-sourced reviews of research (Beatty *et al.* 2009; Bambra 2011; Lindsay and Houston 2011, 2013). However, while our discussion specifically draws upon and confirms the analysis provided by, for example, Lindsay and Houston (2013), there are areas where this article – and much of the evidence presented elsewhere in this Special Issue – offers new insights. First, in this article and elsewhere in this Special Issue, authors have broadened the multi-disciplinary approach to researching the nature of disability claiming and potential policy solutions. We have drawn attention to robust clinical studies that have identified both significant health barriers among those on DBs and apparent progress following well-evidenced clinical interventions. Elsewhere, we have highlighted a broader evidence base on how the workplace and labour market shape opportunities and barriers for people on DBs.

We have also sought to link this expanded discussion of the 'nature of the problem' to a critical evaluation of the current UK policy agenda. We have argued that there is a disconnect between the multi-faceted

17

complexity of the DB problem and the rationale and content of policy, which is rooted in a behaviourist logic and largely relies upon a combination of increased conditionality and work-first activation. Such approaches might reduce on-flow in the short-term – it is self-evident that any determined effort to enhance regulation to restrict DB claiming will reduce the number of successful claims. But it is difficult to see how such policies have any relevance to improving the long-term employability and health (or mitigating the disability-related limitations) of people on DBs. It is therefore unsurprising that job outcomes for people on ESA have been disappointing under the Work Programme, as they were for IB claimants under PtW. It is difficult to arrive at more detailed conclusions about the efficacy of current programmes – the Work Programme's market orientation and black box funding mechanisms mean that programme content is treated as intellectual property, with no incentive to share information on 'what works' (or does not) in assisting people on DBs (Ceolta-Smith *et al.* 2015). Meanwhile, recent gradual reductions in ESA numbers are likely to be the result of measures to restrict access and increase means-testing, rather than positive outcomes from activation measures such as the Work Programme. While those denied benefits may 'not be on ESA in the future, they may not be in employment either' (Lindsay and Houston 2011: 714); and restrictions to DBs combined with other welfare retrenchment policies have clearly caused considerable hardship (Beatty and Fothergill 2015).

We have also seen that alternative policy approaches are possible, but that the UK is not alone in struggling to identify solutions. Denmark has grappled with its own DB problem, but has adopted very different policy responses, rooted in joined-up models of activation and collaboration with employers to facilitate adjustments in the workplace. There are principles in the Danish model – especially the engagement of employers as full partners in assisting people to cope with their conditions – that would appear to be of value in the UK context. However, the continuing high levels of disability claiming in parts of Denmark highlight the limitations of any supply-side policy in addressing the complex combination of issues that trap people on benefits for long periods.

A number of lessons for policy are discernable from the preceding discussion. If individuals are to be assisted into sustainable employment (rather than merely being prevented from claiming DBs) there is a need for well-funded, targeted activation that is flexible enough to deal with the range of employability-related barriers faced by people on DBs. Arriving at a more holistic, evidence-based approach to addressing employability-related barriers will need policymakers to grow out of their fixation with narrow, behaviourist approaches to 'incentivizing' claimants. Meanwhile, current policies to limit benefit uprating and increase the reach of means-testing are less likely to incentivize jobseeking than to increase the risk of poverty among claimants (Beatty and Fothergill 2015) and so further undermine their employability.

People claiming DBs face a range of health and disability-related barriers, which vary in their complexity and severity. Accordingly, there is a need to retain a system that separates out a 'work-related activity group' who can be helped towards a return to work, from those facing the most severe barriers. The establishment of this distinction under ESA was positive in this respect, but there is a need for more sophisticated tools to measure both barriers and work capabilities. Better quality capability measurement can help to inform both health-focused condition management programmes and workplace adjustments that will be needed if we are to assist people to move from welfare to work. Clearly, any assessment of work capacity needs to be based on robust clinical measurement rather than pre-set government targets for removing people from benefits (Harris and Rahilly 2011). Most importantly, policymakers must accept that the vast majority of DB claimants face health and disability-related barriers, and that condition management and occupational health services will be an essential element in helping people to cope with these limitations in the workplace. Condition management interventions piloted under PtW produced mixed outcomes (like most other health services dealing with diverse client groups), but elsewhere in this Special Issue it is argued that the further testing and development of such services may have the potential to contribute to improved employability and health provision (Purdie and Kellett 2015).

There is also a need for such health and employability provision to be joined-up with policies to address the labour market and workplace aspects of the DB problem. Inequalities in the quality and availability of work are crucial to explaining the concentration of DB claiming in post-industrial regions. Demand-side interventions that promote jobs growth will therefore be required to address these inequalities. A further contribution of this article, and others in this Special Issue, is to emphasize the need for workplace interventions. Too many of the jobs that are seen as appropriate destinations for people leaving DBs are in fact defined by content and conditions that are unconducive to managing health and disability-related limitations at work. There is a need for a renewed partnership between the state and employers: the state should incentivize adjustments to the work environment and job content that might facilitate returns-to-work for people on DBs; employers need to play a proactive role in identifying potential adjustments and creating a management culture that assists the reintegration of those managing health conditions or disabilities. The retention of activation targeting a distinctive work-related activity group can *only* be justified if policy also addresses workplace barriers and engages employers as key partners in delivering opportunity. These relatively modest policy prescriptions to some extent reflect the analysis of advocates of a 'social model of disability', who argue that social, economic and workplace institutions explain the disadvantage of people experiencing a range of health problems and disabilities (Patrick 2012). From this perspective, policy solutions must seek the transformation of these disabling institutions, rather than targeting the supposed failings of the individual.

Some may claim that placing condition management and adjustments in the workplace at the heart of policy solutions makes unrealistic

19

demands of employers. But the regional variations in DB numbers are partly explained by the manner in which recruiters in tight labour markets *are already* making informal adjustments to their expectations and job demands. In 'full employment' regions, employers are more likely to recruit people with health or disability-related barriers given the absence of 'slack' in local labour markets (i.e. where nobody else is available, employers are forced to adjust their demands to facilitate the employment of people with health conditions or disabilities). Policymakers should engage with employers to formalize and transfer a culture of flexibility and adjustment across all labour markets and workplaces.

None of the critics of current policy advocates doing nothing to activate those on DBs who could potentially return to work. For Bambra and Smith (2010: 76) 'more passive approaches have often exacerbated the labour market exclusion experienced by people with a disability or chronic illness'. Similarly, Beatty *et al.* (2009: 718) criticize the policy inertia of the 1980s and 1990s that saw all stakeholders 'turn a blind eye to the scale of the issue'. There is a clear need for policy action. Increasing conditionality and means-testing, and compelling DB claimants to participate in work-first activation, may discourage some from claiming benefits – the 'deterrence effect' often celebrated by work-first advocates (for a discussion, see Daguerre and Etherington 2009) – but these measures are unlikely to produce long-term improvements in employability or health. We believe that our review of evidence above, lessons from countries like Denmark, and the findings of research presented elsewhere in this Special Issue, point to the need for a different approach. A renewed commitment to evidence-based policy in this area would produce holistic strategies to address health, employability and labour market-related barriers – the complex and inter-connected factors that explain why too many people in the UK remain trapped on long-term DBs.

## Note

1. Throughout this article 'disability benefits' is used as a generic term to cover the main long-term disability/sickness/'incapacity benefits' claimed by people of working age – previously Incapacity Benefit, Income Support, and the new Employment and Support Allowance introduced from 2008.

## References

Bambra, C. (2011), *Work, Worklessness and the Political Economy of Health*, Oxford: Oxford University Press.

Bambra, C. and Smith, K. (2010), No longer deserving? Sickness benefit reform and the politics of (ill) health, *Critical Public Health*, 20, 1: 71–83.

Baumberg, B. (2014), Fit-for-work – or work fit for disabled people? The role of changing job demands and control in incapacity claims, *Journal of Social Policy*, 43, 2: 289–310.

Baumberg, B. (2015), From impairment to incapacity – educational inequalities in disabled people's ability to work, *Social Policy & Administration*, 49, 2: 182–98.

Barnes, H. and Sissons, P. (2013), Redefining fit for work: welfare reform and the introduction of the Employment Support Allowance. In C. Lindsay and D. Houston (eds), *Disability Benefits, Welfare Reform and Employment Policy*, Basingstoke: Palgrave Macmillan, pp. 72–93.

Beatty, C. and Fothergill, S. (1994), Registered and hidden unemployment in areas of chronic industrial decline: the case of the UK coalfields. In S. Hardy, G. Lloyd and I. Cundell (eds), *Tackling Unemployment and Social Exclusion: Problems for Regions, Solutions for People*, London: Regional Studies Association, pp. 38–48.

Beatty, C. and Fothergill, S. (2015), Disability benefits in an era of austerity, *Social Policy & Administration*, 49, 2: 161–81.

Beatty, C., Fothergill, S. and Houston, D. (2013), The impact of the UK's disability benefit reforms. In C. Lindsay and D. Houston (eds), *Disability Benefits, Welfare Reform and Employment Policy*, Basingstoke: Palgrave Macmillan, pp. 134–52.

Beatty, C., Fothergill, S. and Macmillan, R. (2000), A theory of employment, unemployment and sickness, *Regional Studies*, 34, 7: 617–30.

Beatty, C., Fothergill, S., Houston, D., Powell, R. and Sissons, P. (2009), A gendered theory of employment, unemployment and sickness, *Environment and Planning C: Government and Policy*, 27, 6: 958–74.

Beatty, C., Fothergill, S., Houston, D., Powell, R. and Sissons, P. (2010), Bringing Incapacity Benefit numbers down: to what extent do women need a different approach? *Policy Studies*, 31, 2: 143–62.

Brix Pedersen, K. (2013), *Replacing Disability Pension for Young People Under 40 with a Rehabilitation Model*, Paper given at the OECD Mental Health and Work Seminar, OECD Headquarters, Paris, France, 17 April.

Carter, B., Danford, A., Howcroft, D., Richardson, H., Smith, A. and Taylor, P. (2013), Stressed out of my box: employee experiences of lean working and occupational ill-health in clerical work in the UK public sector, *Work, Employment & Society*, 27, 5: 747–67.

Centre for Social Justice (CSJ) (2009), *Dynamic Benefits*, London: CSJ.

Ceolta-Smith, J., Salway, S. and Tod, A. (2015), A review of health-related support provision within the UK Work Programme – what's on the menu? *Social Policy & Administration*, 49, 2: 254–76.

Daguerre, A. with Etherington, D. (2009), *Active Labour Market Policies in International Context: What Works Best? Lessons for the UK*, London: Department for Work and Pensions.

Department for Work and Pensions (DWP) (2010), *21st Century Welfare*, London: Department for Work and Pensions.

Dixon, J. and Warrener, M. (2008), *Pathways to Work: Qualitative Study of In-Work Support, DWP Research Report No. 478*, Leeds: Corporate Document Services.

Easterlow, D. and Smith, S. J. (2003), Health and employment: towards a New Deal, *Policy and Politics*, 31, 4: 511–33.

Etherington, D. and Ingold, J. (2012), Welfare to work and the inclusive labour market: a comparative study of activation policies for sickness benefit claimants in the UK and Denmark, *Journal of European Social Policy*, 22, 1: 30–44.

Garthwaite, K. (2015), 'Keeping meself to meself' – how social networks can influence narratives of stigma and identity for long-term sickness benefits recipients, *Social Policy & Administration*, 49, 2: 199–212.

Garthwaite, K., Bambra, C., Warren, J., Kasim, A. and Greig, G. (2014), Shifting the goalposts: a longitudinal mixed-methods study of the health of long-term Incapacity Benefit Recipients during a period of substantial change to the UK social security system, *Journal of Social Policy*, 43, 2: 311–30.

Grammenos, S. (2011), *Indicators of Disability Equality in Europe*, Leeds: Academic Network of European Disability Experts.

Grant, A. (2013), Welfare reform, conditionality and targets: Jobcentre Plus advisers' experiences of targets and sanctions, *Journal of Poverty and Social Justice*, 21, 2: 165–76.

Green, A. (1994), The changing structure, distribution and spatial segregation of the unemployed and economically inactive in Great Britain, *Geoforum*, 26, 4: 373–94.

Green, A. and Shuttleworth, I. (2010), Local differences, perceptions and incapacity benefit claimants: implications for policy delivery, *Policy Studies*, 31, 2: 223–43.

Green, A. and Shuttleworth, I. (2013), Are incapacity benefit claimants beyond employment? Exploring issues of employability. In C. Lindsay and D. Houston (eds), *Disability Benefits, Welfare Reform and Employment Policy*, Basingstoke: Palgrave Macmillan, pp. 54–71.

Harrington, M. (2010), *An Independent Review of the Work Capability Assessment*, London: Stationery Office.

Harris, N. and Rahilly, S. (2011), Extra capacity in the labour market? ESA and activation for the sick and disabled in the UK. In S. Devetzi and S. Stendahl (eds), *Too Sick to Work?*, Alphen aan den Rijn: Kluwer, pp. 43–75.

House of Commons Work and Pensions Committee (HoC) (2013), *Can the Work Programme Work for All User Groups? Report HC162*, London: The Stationery Office.

Jones, A., Rice, N. and Roberts, J. (2010), Sick of work or too sick to work? Evidence on self-reported health shocks and early retirement from the BHPS, *Economic Modelling*, 27: 866–80.

Kellett, S., Bickerstaff, D., Purdie, F., Dyke, A., Filer, S., Lomax, V. and Tomlinson, H. (2011), The clinical and occupational effectiveness of condition management for Incapacity Benefit recipients, *British Journal of Clinical Psychology*, 50, 2: 164–77.

Kemp, P. A. and Davidson, J. (2009), Gender differences among new claimants of Incapacity Benefit, *Journal of Social Policy*, 38, 4: 589–606.

Kemp, P. A. and Davidson, J. (2010), Employability trajectories among new claimants of Incapacity Benefit, *Policy Studies*, 31, 2: 203–21.

Kjeldsen, M., Houlberg, H. and Hodelund, J. (2013), *Handicap og Beskæftigelse. Udviklingen Mellem 2002 og 2012*, Copenhagen: The Danish National Centre for Social Research.

Larsen, F. (2013), Active labour market reform in Denmark: the role of governance in policy change. In E. Z. Brodkin and G. Marston (eds), *Work and the Welfare State: Street-level Organizations and Workfare Politics*, Copenhagen: DJOF.

Lindsay, C. and Dutton, M. (2013), Promoting healthy routes to employability: lessons for welfare-to-work in the UK, *Policy and Politics*, 41, 2: 183–200.

Lindsay, C. and Houston, D. (2011), Fit for purpose? Welfare reform and challenges for health and labour market policy in the UK, *Environment and Planning A*, 43, 3: 703–21.

Lindsay, C. and Houston, D. (2013), *Disability Benefits, Welfare Reform and Employment Policy*, Basingstoke: Palgrave Macmillan.

Lindsay, C. and McQuaid, R. W. (2009), New governance and the case of activation policies: comparing experiences in Denmark and the Netherlands, *Social Policy & Administration*, 43, 5: 445–63.

McKee-Ryan, F. M., Song, Z., Wamberg, C. R. and Kinicki, A. J. (2005), Psychological and physical well-being during unemployment: a meta-analytic study, *Journal of Applied Psychology*, 90, 1: 53–76.

National Audit Office (NAO) (2010), *Support to Incapacity Benefits Claimants Through Pathways to Work*, London: NAO.

Organisation for Economic Co-operation and Development (OECD) (2011), *Sick on the Job? Myths and Realities about Mental Health at Work*, Paris: OECD.

Organisation for Economic Co-operation and Development (OECD) (2013), *Employment Outlook*, Paris: OECD.

Patrick, R. (2012), All in it together? Disabled people, the Coalition and welfare to work, *Journal of Poverty and Social Justice*, 20, 3: 307–22.

Purdie, F. and Kellett, S. (2015), The influence of presenting health condition on eventual return to work for individuals receiving health-related welfare benefits, *Social Policy & Administration*, 49, 2: 236–53.

Rees, J., Whitworth, A. and Carter, E. (2014), Support for all in the UK Work Programme? Differential payments, same old problem, *Social Policy & Administration*, 48, 2: 221–39.

Rick, J., Carroll, C., Jagger, N. and Hillage, J. (2008), *Review of the Effectiveness and Cost Effectiveness of Interventions, Strategies, Programmes and Policies to Help Recipients of Incapacity Benefits Return to Employment (Paid and Unpaid)*, Brighton: Institute for Employment Studies.

Robroek, S., Schuring, M., Croezen, S., Stattin, M. and Burdorf, A. (2013), Poor health, unhealthy behaviors and unfavorable work characteristics influence pathways of exit from paid employment among older workers in Europe: a four year follow-up study, *Scandinavian Journal of Work and Environment Health*, 39, 1: 125–33.

Shildrick, T., MacDonald, R., Webster, C. and Garthwaite, K. (2012), *Poverty and Insecurity: Life in Low-pay, No-pay Britain*, Bristol: Policy Press.

Taylor, P., Cunningham, I., Newsome, K. and Scholarios, D. (2010), Too scared to go sick – reformulating the research agenda on sickness absence, *Industrial Relations Journal*, 41, 4: 270–88.

Webster, D., Brown, J., Macdonald, E. and Turok, I. (2013), The interaction of health, labour market conditions and long-term sickness benefit claims in a post-industrial city: a Glasgow case study. In C. Lindsay and D. Houston (eds), *Disability Benefits, Welfare Reform and Employment Policy*, Basingstoke: Palgrave Macmillan, pp. 111–33.

Whittaker, W. and Sutton, M. (2015), Measuring the impacts of health conditions on work incapacity – evidence from the British Household Panel Survey, *Social Policy & Administration*, 49, 2: 213–35.

**2**

*Disability Benefits in an Age of Austerity*

**Christina Beatty and Steve Fothergill**

## Introduction

The UK has a disability benefits crisis. The scale of the problem took some while to be recognized, first by labour market analysts and benefits administrators and only much later by politicians and the general public. But continuously since the late 1990s the number of men and women out-of-work claiming disability benefits in the UK has hovered around the 2.5 million mark. This represents more than 6 per cent of the entire working age population. The UK's disability claimant rate places it well towards the higher end by international standards (Kemp 2006).

This article considers disability benefits in the UK in the era of welfare reform and fiscal austerity that followed the financial crisis of 2008. In order to do so, it first takes a long-view of the rise in disability claimant numbers and explains how and why this came about, drawing on both theory and empirical evidence. This assessment is then deployed to help anticipate the new trends that are likely to emerge as welfare reform and fiscal austerity work their way through the benefits system. The article's distinctive contribution is that it synthesizes insights from a range of previous studies of UK disability claimants, including the authors' substantial research in this field, and brings this accumulated knowledge and understanding to bear in assessing likely trends and impacts in the near future.

## Defining 'disability benefits'

It is helpful to begin by clarifying terminology. The term 'disability benefits' is used here to describe a family of UK welfare benefits comprising Incapacity Benefit, Income Support and National Insurance (NI) credits paid on the grounds of disability, Severe Disablement Allowance, and Employment and Support Allowance (ESA). Since 2008, a process of

*New Perspectives on Health, Disability, Welfare and the Labour Market*, First Edition.
Edited by Colin Lindsay, Bent Greve, Ignazio Cabras, Nick Ellison and Stephen Kellett.
© 2015 John Wiley & Sons, Ltd. Published 2015 by John Wiley & Sons, Ltd.

reform has been underway and the aim is that by 2015 all qualifying disability claimants will have moved onto ESA. The intention is also that by 2018 all ESA claimants who claim means-tested benefits will in turn have moved across onto Universal Credit, which is planned to replace most working-age benefits, though the rules applying to ESA claimants will stay substantially unchanged so they will remain a distinct sub-group within the benefits system. In the UK context, the term 'disability benefits', as defined here, is often used interchangeably with 'incapacity benefits' to describe the same group of welfare benefits.

To qualify for one or other of these disability benefits, a claimant normally has to be aged between 16 and state pension age (65 for men and currently rising in stages from 60 to 65 for women). They also have to be out-of-work. The exceptions are a very small number of claimants above state pension age who carry on working but are entitled to claim disability benefits for a short while if they fall ill, and a small number of individuals with health problems or disabilities who undertake 'permitted work' as part of a rehabilitation programme. All disability claimants have to demonstrate a sufficient degree of ill health or disability to be not required to look for work as a condition of their benefit entitlement.

In the UK, disability benefit claimants are an entirely separate group from the unemployed claiming Jobseeker's Allowance, who are required to look for work. It is not possible to claim disability and unemployment benefits at the same time. Also, 'disability benefits' as defined here do not include a further benefit known as Disability Living Allowance (DLA), intended to help offset the additional costs of disability. DLA is claimed by approaching 3 million people but eligibility is not restricted to just the out-of-work and it can be claimed by men and women above state pension age and by parents in respect of disabled children.

One of the reasons that the huge numbers out-of-work on disability benefits are a major problem is that they represent a massive waste of talent and productive potential. In an age of fiscal austerity they are also a major drain on the UK Exchequer. It is impossible to pin down the full cost because entitlement to disability benefits often brings entitlement to other benefits in its wake. Income Support, for example, can be claimed as a means-tested top-up. Nearly half of all disability claimants claim Housing Benefit, half claim Council Tax Benefit, and almost half also claim DLA (Beatty *et al.* 2009). In turn, these entitlements can lead to further passported benefits such as free school meals, free prescriptions and free dental care.

Bearing in mind that in 2012–13 the forecast expenditure on ESA and Incapacity Benefit alone was just short of £10 billion (HM Treasury 2013), it would not be unreasonable to suppose that the full financial cost to the UK Exchequer of disability benefit claimants is of the order of £15 billion to £20 billion a year. This equates to £6,000–£8,000 per claimant per year, or £120–£160 a week. These figures put into context the UK Government's desire to bring down disability claimant numbers

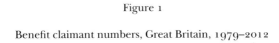

Figure 1

Benefit claimant numbers, Great Britain, 1979–2012

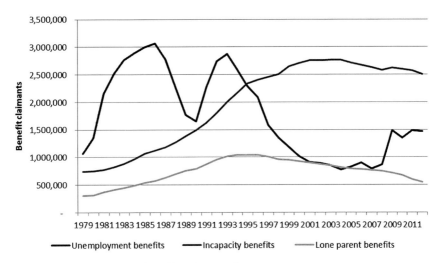

*Source:* Department for Work and Pensions, various years.

and spending at a time when the political priority is to reduce the scale of the budget deficit.

## The Rise in Disability Claimant Numbers

### Overall trends

Figure 1 shows disability claimant numbers in Great Britain between 1979 and 2012, alongside the numbers claiming unemployment benefits and lone parent benefits. The figure illustrates very well why disability benefits have become such a policy concern. Since the end of the 1970s, the numbers out-of-work claiming disability benefits have tripled. The numbers claiming unemployment benefits, by contrast, remain well below peak levels in the 1980s and early 1990s. The numbers claiming lone parent benefits have also halved since the mid-1990s.

The trends through time in figure 1 reflect changing benefit rules as well as underlying trends in the labour market and economy. A substantial proportion of the fall in claimant unemployment numbers since the mid-1990s, for example, reflects tighter rules on eligibility: the numbers now recorded as unemployed by the UK Government's Labour Force Survey are around a million higher than the claimant count. Likewise, eligibility for lone parent benefits has been reduced in stages, from parents of under-16s to parents of under-fives only. Nevertheless, the upshot

27

is that disability claimants now constitute by far the largest group of out-of-work claimants of working age.

The big increase in disability claimant numbers began in the 1980s, from a base of well below 1 million. By the early 1990s, the numbers were reaching 2 million and there were the first attempts to stem the increase. The year 1995 is a significant date in the story because it saw the replacement of what was then Invalidity Benefit by Incapacity Benefit, with rather less generous entitlements. The 1995 reforms also introduced a new medical test – the Personal Capability Assessment – carried out early in the claim by doctors working on behalf of the government to supplement the initial medical sign-off by the claimant's own doctor. After 1995, the pace of increase in disability claimant numbers began to slow. Disability claimant numbers peaked at over 2.7 million in 2003.

What is striking is that, across Britain as a whole, disability claimant numbers did not fall significantly during the long period of economic growth from 1993 to 2008. A modest fall of around 200,000 occurred only during the final stages, from 2003 to 2008. Since 2009 there has been a further gradual reduction which is without doubt attributable to welfare reform, discussed later. What the resistance of claimant numbers to fall during a period of sustained economic growth illustrates is the extent to which many disability claimants had become marginalized from the rest of the UK workforce. Indeed, statistics from the Department for Work and Pensions (DWP) show that the modest fall in the headline total after 2003 was entirely due to a reduction in on-flows to disability benefits, as fewer people with health problems or disabilities lost their jobs or failed to find alternative work (National Audit Office 2010). By contrast, off-flows of existing claimants from disability benefits remained at a largely unchanged and low level.

*Gender*

Figure 2 disaggregates the increase in disability claimant numbers between men and women. It also takes an even longer view, extending back to the early 1960s. However, changes over the years in the way that short-term claimants have been handled within the benefits system mean that the data here refers only to working-age disability claimants of six months or more. These are, nevertheless, the vast majority of disability claimants.

The number of women claiming disability benefits has been consistently below the number of men. Partly, this reflects benefit rules: men on disability benefits move across onto a state pension at the age of 65, whereas until 2010 women did so at the age of 60. There has therefore been a group of 60–64-year-old men in receipt of disability benefits for which there has, until very recently, been no corresponding group of women. But there is also evidence in figure 2 that the increase in disability claims among women took off rather later – in the 1990s rather than the 1980s. The reduction in the number of claimants since 2003

Figure 2

Male and female disability claimants* (6 months+), Great Britain, 1963–2012

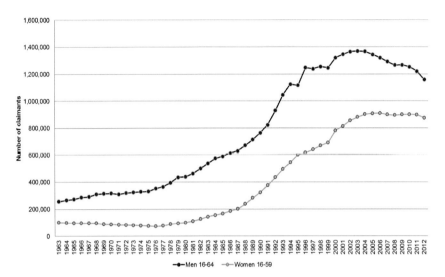

*Source:* Webster 2004, and updates by authors based on Department for Work and Pensions, various years.

*Note:* * = excluding Severe Disablement Allowance.

has also been almost exclusively among men. The effect has been to create a more even gender balance. Indeed, between 1984 and 2008 the ratio between 16–59-year-old men and women claiming disability benefits shifted from 61:39 in favour of men to just 52:48 (Beatty *et al.* 2010). Age for age, women are now almost as likely to claim disability benefits as men.

## Geography

Figure 3 shows the disability benefit claimant rate by local authority district across Great Britain in August 2012. The data here is expressed as a percentage of all adults between the ages of 16 and 64. There are substantial differences between places.

For those familiar with the geography of Britain, it will be immediately apparent that the highest claimant rates, approaching or above 10 per cent, are mostly found in Britain's older industrial areas – in the South Wales Valleys, in the North of England in places such as Merseyside, Lancashire, South Yorkshire, Teesside, Durham and Tyneside, and in the West of Scotland in and around Glasgow. These are the parts of Britain where large-scale industrial job losses occurred in the 1980s and

29

Figure 3

Disability benefit claimant rate by district, Great Britain, August 2012

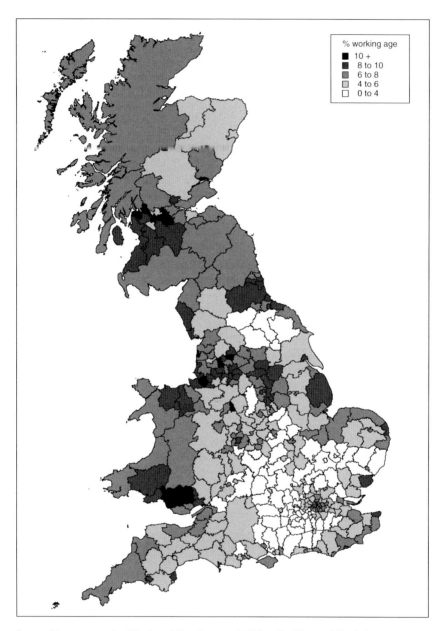

% working age
- 10 +
- 8 to 10
- 6 to 8
- 4 to 6
- 0 to 4

*Sources:* Department for Work and Pensions and Office for National Statistics.

early 1990s, and where there has been a continuing imbalance between labour demand and supply.

Closer scrutiny also highlights a number of seaside towns that have high claimant rates. In southern England these include Great Yarmouth, Tendring district in Essex (which includes Clacton), Thanet in Kent (Margate), Hastings, Weymouth and Torbay. Further north, Blackpool, Scarborough and East Lindsey in Lincolnshire (Skegness) also stand out. Not all seaside towns have high disability claimant rates, but those that are generally regarded as having weaker local economies certainly do.

By contrast, the disability claimant rate in much of southern and eastern England is consistently low – generally below 4 per cent. This is the part of Britain where the economy is strongest and where unemployment problems have traditionally been modest. A group of mainly rural districts in North Yorkshire also have low disability claimant rates – this is a part of the country that on a range of socio-economic indicators has, for some while, looked closer to prosperous southern England than to surrounding areas in the North.

The London boroughs mostly have higher disability claimant rates than surrounding areas, but still much lower rates than much of the North, Scotland and Wales. The rates are highest in parts of Inner, East and North London, pointing to a degree of residential segregation between rich and poor areas across the capital.

Although the differences in disability claimant rates across Britain remain very large, they are actually smaller than at their peak in the late 1990s and early 2000s (McVicar 2013). The modest reduction in overall disability claimant numbers from 2003 onwards occurred mostly in the high-claimant areas, where the reduction was, in some cases, as large as one-quarter or one-third. This may owe something to a 'cohort effect', as claimants from the earlier era of industrial restructuring finally reached pension age. It may also reflect greater competition for jobs from healthy in-migrants in some of Britain's more prosperous local economies, where similar reductions in disability claimant numbers did not occur. The evidence is that where disability numbers fell fastest, economic growth rather than policy intervention was the main driver (Webster *et al.* 2010). In at least one city (Glasgow), improvements in health also appear to have played a role (Webster *et al.* 2013).

## Profile of Claimants

DWP administrative data provides a basic profile of disability claimants. We note above, from this data, that disability claimants are now almost as likely to be women as men. Another clear observation is that the probability of claiming disability benefits rises with age.

The DWP data shows that a high proportion of disability claimants have been claiming these benefits for a very long time. The up-to-date statistical picture on the duration of claims is complicated by the changeover from Incapacity Benefit (and associated benefits) to

ESA. But the data does tell us that in 2007, before the changeover started, around 55 per cent of disability claimants had been in receipt of these benefits for five years or more, and around three-quarters for more than two years. This is a stark contrast with the unemployed on Jobseeker's Allowance, for whom claims are typically of much shorter duration.

The DWP data also provides an insight into claimants' health problems or disabilities. The data records the primary medical reason for allowing the disability claim; in practice, a great many claimants suffer from more than one health problem or disability (Kemp and Davidson 2010). According to the data for 2012, the primary reason for entitlement to ESA for 43 per cent of claimants is 'mental or behavioural problems'. This is a broad category, spanning stress and depression through to much more tightly defined psychological problems. The category also includes drug and alcohol problems. The second most numerous category, accounting for 15 per cent of ESA claimants, covers those with 'musculoskeletal problems'.

Over the years, the proportion of disability claimants recorded as having mental or behavioural problems has risen, while the proportion with musculoskeletal problems has declined. The changing balance partly reflects a generational shift: a group of men made redundant from heavy industry in the 1980s and 1990s, who had often picked up physical injuries over the course of the working lives, have been passing out of the figures into retirement to be replaced by a more diverse group of both men and women with different work histories. There have also been changes in the way the medical profession approaches back pain – a key musculoskeletal problem – with activity rather than rest now recommended as the treatment. Beyond the two big groups of 'mental or behavioural' and 'musculoskeletal', other specific illnesses or disabilities account for much smaller numbers, generally less than 5 per cent of ESA claimants.

A survey of more than 3,500 disability claimants across eight local areas around Britain (Beatty et al. 2009) found that illness or injury is cited by more than 70 per cent of disability claimants as the principal reason for their last job coming to an end. For many, a specific event, such as injury or a deterioration in health, triggered job loss and they have subsequently not returned to work. Only around a quarter of disability claimants say they 'can't do any work' but the remainder nearly all report health limitations on their ability to work. Typically, there are certain types of work that claimants no longer feel able to do (e.g. heavy labour) or limitations on how much work they feel able to undertake. Around half expect their health problems or disabilities to get worse; only 5 per cent expect to get better.

It is therefore not surprising that health problems shape the way that disability claimants see their prospects. The same survey data shows that only around a third would like a job, now or further into the future. In more than 90 per cent of cases the reason given for not wanting a job is that their health is not good enough. Even among those who would like a job, 90 per cent cite ill health, injury or disability as an obstacle to finding work, and three-quarters say they think employers would regard them as 'too ill or disabled' or 'too big a risk'.

But ill health and/or disability are not the only defining features of disability claimants. The same survey data underlines the extent to which they are a poorly-qualified group with mostly lower-grade manual work experience. Some 60 per cent report that they had 'no formal qualifications', and some 80 per cent of women and 85 per cent of men had usually worked in manual occupations.

On the other hand, it is important not to characterize disability claimants as men and women who have rarely, or never, been in paid employment. In the same survey, just 9 per cent of women and 6 per cent of men said they had never had a job. Substantial and often continuous work experience is common: one-third of men and one-quarter of women reported that they had been in their last job for 20 years or more.

## Explaining the Increase

Drawing on empirical evidence from the UK, Beatty *et al.* (2000) argued that disability benefit claims are best understood as part of a triangular relationship between the levels of employment, unemployment and sickness. In particular, they argued that job loss can lead to increases in recorded sickness (i.e. disability benefit claims) as well as to increases in recorded unemployment, even if there is no change in the underlying health of the population. They also argued that welfare rules – for example, qualifying criteria and differences in payment rates – help to allocate claimants between disability benefits and other benefits.

More recently, Lindsay and Houston (2013) have argued that disability claims in the UK and elsewhere are best understood as reflecting the interaction of labour markets, ill health and employability. Their view is that difficult labour local markets, ill health and/or disability, and poor skills and qualifications combine to marginalize some men and women from paid employment, and that because of their ill health they claim disability rather than unemployment benefits.

These are not two rival theories. They are in fact entirely compatible and, in many respects, two different ways of expressing and explaining the same processes. A narrative of the increase in disability claims in the UK can usefully draw on elements of both.

The starting points need to be, first, that ill health and disability are actually quite widespread in the working age population, and second, that they are not necessarily an absolute bar to working. The UK's Labour Force Survey for 2012, for example, identifies 8.3 million adults of working age who are disabled (in terms of the Disability Discrimination Act 1995) or report a work-limiting illness or disability – around one in five of the whole working age population. Of these, 4.1 million, or 49 per cent, are in employment. This is well below the employment rate among men and women without health problems or disabilities

(76 per cent) but it illustrates the point that ill health or disability is not always an insurmountable obstacle to holding down a job.

Beatty *et al.* (2000) described the ill health and disability among those in work or recorded as unemployed as 'hidden sickness', in that it is not reflected in disability benefit numbers. However, they argued that when job loss occurs, this hidden sickness begins to become 'visible': men and women with health problems or disabilities are often among those that employers prefer to shed, retaining instead the fit and healthy with fewer constraints on the work they can undertake, and some of the men and women with health problems volunteer themselves for redundancy because of the difficulties they face carrying on working.

This is what began to happen in the early 1980s, a period of immense job loss in the UK especially from manufacturing and mining in the North of England, Scotland and Wales. At first, it was often the newly redundant industrial workers themselves – the ex-miners and ex-steelworkers for example – who moved onto disability benefits. They accessed disability benefits rather than unemployment benefits because they carried forward ill health and injuries from their former employment and because they were mostly financially better off doing so. The recession at the beginning of the 1990s added a further wave of job losses.

One of the earliest examples to be documented showed how in the UK's coalmining areas the principal labour market adjustment in response to the loss of mining jobs was an increase in recorded 'permanent sickness' rather than in recorded unemployment (Beatty and Fothergill 1996). This observation helped provoke extensive discussion of the scale of 'hidden unemployment' on disability benefits (Armstrong 1999; Fieldhouse and Hollywood 1999; MacKay 1999; Webster 2002; Bell and Smith 2004; McVicar 2006, 2008; Little 2007).

That neither the short-lived economic boom in the second half of the 1980s nor the first stages of recovery from the early 1990s recession resulted in falling disability numbers is not surprising. Labour markets take time to adjust fully in response to job loss. The rising numbers on disability benefits in the 1980s and 1990s were made up of not just those who had made been redundant from mining and manufacturing, but also those in poor health who subsequently lost out in the normal competition for jobs.

Wherever there is an imbalance between labour demand and labour supply, ill health or disability is one of the great discriminators determining exactly which individuals are able to secure and maintain employment. Other things being equal, employers prefer the fit and healthy. Indeed, over the years they have probably become *less* tolerant of sickness absences, partly because fewer men and women with health problems remain in work (a corollary of the increase in disability claimant numbers) and partly because many organizations, notably in the public sector, have become more adept at monitoring absences and setting targets.

34

Poor qualifications, low skills, low-grade work experience, advancing age and low motivation tend to be the other discriminators that determine which individuals find and maintain employment. Where an individual faces more than one of these obstacles – which can often be the case with disability claimants – their chances of finding work can be slim. In a period of economic recovery, the numbers claiming unemployment benefits also fall more quickly because the unemployed claimants, unlike their counterparts on disability benefits, are required to look for work and thereby stay in touch with the labour market.

That the final stages of the long period of economic growth up to 2008 did not lead to bigger reductions in disability claimant numbers came as more of a surprise. Beatty *et al.* (2000) had predicted that once claimant unemployment reached historically low levels, further economic growth might be expected to erode the number claiming disability benefits. This happened to only a marginal extent, as figure 1 shows. The disengagement of so many disability claimants from the labour market, documented in Beatty *et al.* (2009), is likely to be a key reason why disability numbers did not fall further during this era of economic growth. But in addition this was also a period when there was a surge in international in-migration to the UK, providing an alternative source of labour supply. Once more, fit and healthy workers (in this instance from abroad) were preferred to those with ill health or disability.

In the parts of the UK worst affected by job losses in the 1980s and early 1990s, the long economic recovery never did plug the gap between labour demand and supply. With a continuing imbalance in these local labour markets it was therefore inevitable that some individuals would be squeezed out and, in a competitive labour market, it has been those who are least able or least willing to keep a foothold in paid employment who have been marginalized. These men and women are typically the poorly qualified, low-skilled manual workers in poor health, whose alternative would at best be unrewarding work at or close to the national minimum wage.

Competition in the labour market also explains why so many women now claim disability benefits and why they are concentrated in the same places as men. The industrial job losses that first triggered the rise in disability claims impacted disproportionately on men. The textiles and clothing industries, which have together shed over a million jobs in the UK since the 1960s, were once huge employers of women, but many other parts of mining and manufacturing were traditionally male-dominated. Steel, shipbuilding, heavy engineering and the motor industry are good examples. However, in the parts of Britain where disability claimant rates are highest – often older industrial areas – high claimant rates are found among both men and women (Beatty *et al.* 2009).

The explanation lies in the fact that far fewer jobs are now seen as exclusively 'male' or 'female'. So while the men made redundant a generation ago from industries such as coal, steel and shipbuilding might have shunned what they saw as 'women's work', their sons have rarely had the same luxury. The old industries have often gone, while the requirement to look for work as a condition of benefit receipt, and the impact of government schemes such as the Work Programme mean that it is not easy to remain on Jobseeker's Allowance for extended periods. So, a younger group of men who a generation ago would have found jobs in industry have, instead, taken up employment in shops, hotels, catering, hospitals and offices, often in roles that once might have been filled by women. In doing so, they have made the labour market in the places they live more difficult for women. Many of the women who fail to find work have then ended up claiming benefits, including disability benefits, in the same way as their male counterparts. In this way, unemployment is transmitted from men to women in the places where there are not enough jobs for everyone (Beatty et al. 2009).

For the men and women excluded from employment in this way, disability benefits have hitherto offered a more attractive way forward than Jobseeker's Allowance. Disability benefits have been a little more generous and, for those with sufficient recent NI credits, disability benefits have until recently not been means-tested, unlike Jobseeker's Allowance which has always been means-tested for longer-term claimants. This meant that for many claimants, disability benefits could be combined with other sources of household income, such as a partner in work. On disability benefits there has also been no requirement to look for work – work that anyway may be unattractive, low-paid and (bearing in mind issues of age, health and poor qualifications) difficult to obtain. Men and women with ill health or disability have normally been entitled to disability benefits and they have therefore almost always claimed them in preference to unemployment benefits.

Added to this, the effect of lengthening durations on disability benefits saps the enthusiasm of many to re-engage with the labour market. Long-term claimants adjust their lifestyle and aspirations to fit with the diminished job opportunities they perceive to be available, lowering their standards of consumption to fit with reduced household income. Their 'fitness to work' often declines as despondency sets in, and disabilities worsen with age. An initial willingness to consider new employment is thus gradually replaced by a complete detachment from the world of work, rationalized in terms of largely insurmountable health obstacles.

None of this indicates that the health problems and disabilities affecting the men and women who claim disability benefits are anything less than real, or that the older industrial areas where disability claimant rates are highest do not have higher underlying levels of ill health. What is happening is that in places where there is a surplus of labour, employers have less incentive to hold on to staff in poor health. Once an individual with ill health or disability has lost his or her job, in a difficult local labour market that person is also less likely to find a way back into work.

So although ill health or disability is rarely an absolute obstacle to employment, even in the eyes of disability claimants themselves, in practice even modest incapacities can prove to be a formidable obstacle, especially if an individual has no special qualifications or training to offer. By contrast, where there are plenty of jobs – a situation that characterizes much of southern England – large numbers of men and women with health problems or disabilities do not hang around on disability benefits. They either stay in work or, if they lose their job, find new work.

In other words, the UK's high incapacity claimant numbers are, as Lindsay and Houston (2013) argue, an issue of *jobs, health* and *employability*. But they also need to be understood, as Beatty *et al.* (2000) argue, as part of a triangular relationship between *employment, unemployment* and *sickness*.

## Welfare Reform

For more than a decade there has been a political consensus in the UK that the numbers on disability benefits need to be brought down. The pre-2010 Labour Government's initial efforts, through its New Deal for Disabled People and later the Pathways to Work scheme, were focused on providing additional support to claimants to re-engage with the labour market. Most new claimants were mandated to engage with these support services, whereas existing claimants opted-in on a voluntary basis. From 2006 onwards, however, Labour began to introduce reforms to the disability benefits themselves (DWP 2006, 2008). This process has continued under the post-2010 coalition Government. As a result, four key reforms have been simultaneously underway in the first half of the 2010s.

The first is the application of a tougher medical test – the Work Capability Assessment – as the gateway to the new ESA. This was introduced by Labour and has applied to all new disability claimants since October 2008. The Work Capability Assessment takes place three rather than six months into a claim. It uses a points-based system and examines what activities the claimant is capable of undertaking. If the claimant scores sufficiently highly, he or she qualifies for ESA. The initial expectation, based on a pilot study, was that around 12 per cent of the claimants who qualified for Incapacity Benefit under the old medical test would not qualify for ESA under the Work Capability Assessment (DWP 2007). In practice, the failure rate has proved much higher. The effect of the tougher medical test is that the gateway to disability benefits has narrowed.

The second reform, the re-testing of existing claimants, was also introduced by Labour, although it was not part of its initial plans for ESA. The intention is that by 2014 all pre-2008 disability claimants will be called in for the new medical test. They will then be routed onto ESA or, if they fail to qualify, onto other benefits such as Jobseeker's Allowance or (if they fail to qualify again) out of the benefits system altogether. The re-testing of existing claimants was piloted in two areas in late 2010 and early 2011. From April 2011 re-testing was rolled out nationally, with the number of tests carried out each week gradually ramping up.

The third reform, the introduction of a new requirement to engage in work-related activity, is another Labour measure. All those who qualify for ESA are allocated to one of two groups – a Support Group, who are deemed to have sufficiently serious health problems or disabilities to receive unconditional support, and a Work-related Activity Group, for whom ESA comes with strings attached. All claimants in this second group are required to attend work-focused interviews, initially at monthly intervals, at which they are advised on steps to find suitable work including training, voluntary work or job placement for a few hours a week, or physical or mental rehabilitation. Advisers then draw up an 'action plan' to which claimants are expected to adhere. Failure to engage in the work-related interviews runs the risk of benefit sanctions. The underpinning assumption is that, for the Work-related Activity Group, ESA should only be a temporary benefit, pending the claimant's return to work.

The fourth reform, the time limiting of entitlement to non-means tested benefit, is an addition by the coalition Government. Incapacity Benefit, now in the process of being replaced by ESA, was never means-tested except for a small number of post-2002 claimants with significant income from a personal or company pension. This meant that other sources of household income – a partner's earnings for example – were not docked off a claimant's financial entitlement. However, from April 2012 onwards there has been a 12-month limit on the duration of non-means tested ESA for those in the Work-related Activity Group. After the expiry of the 12 months, these claimants are only eligible for the means-tested version of ESA.

## Impact of the Reforms

### Shifting the boundaries

The main impact of the reforms to disability benefits is to shift where individuals are placed within the UK benefits system. The reforms impact sequentially. The new medical test to access ESA has been up-and-running for new claimants for some while, and there is also growing experience of its retrospective application to existing claimants. By contrast, the time-limiting of non-means tested entitlement begins only after 12 months on ESA, and only from 2012 onwards, so there is less hard evidence on outcomes. On time-limiting, it is necessary to rely more heavily on the DWP's forecasts.

The principal effect of the new medical test on *new claimants* is to reduce the on-flow to ESA compared to its predecessor benefits. Based on data for 2010 and 2011, Beatty and Fothergill (2011) estimated the reduced on-flow as being around 45,000 a year, or a cumulative total of around 140,000 over the 2011–14 period. The DWP estimates that 50 per cent of the claimants who fail to qualify for ESA will go on to claim Jobseeker's Allowance instead, 20 per cent will move onto another benefit (e.g. Income Support as a lone parent or Carer's Allowance) and 30 per cent will move off benefit entirely (DWP 2011a).

The effect of the new medical test on *existing claimants* can be gauged from data on the re-assessments (DWP 2013: table 11). Of the 700,000 claimants for whom reassessment was completed between October 2010 and August 2012, 30 per cent were placed in the Support Group, 41 per cent in the Work-related Activity Group and 29 per cent (just over 200,000) found 'fit for work' and therefore denied ESA. Beatty and Fothergill (2011) estimated that when the process of reassessment is completed, the final number of existing claimants losing entitlement to disability benefits as a result of re-testing would be 410,000. This estimate was based on data for the pilot areas. The actual figure, based on the more recent DWP figures, seems likely to be close.

Among the claimants losing entitlement, a reasonable assumption based on the DWP figures for those refused ESA would again be that 50 per cent (around 200,000) will claim Jobseeker's Allowance instead, 20 per cent (80,000) will move onto another benefit, and 30 per cent (120,000) will move off benefit entirely.

The large number moved off benefit entirely does not presume that these individuals find employment, although some will do so. Rather, it reflects the fact that having lost (or, in the case of new claimants, failed to gain) entitlement to disability benefit, many men and women will also find that they are not entitled to other means-tested benefits such as Jobseeker's Allowance. Because the means-testing is undertaken on a household basis, other sources of household income – a partner in work for example – or significant household savings will disqualify them.

The effect of the new medical test is therefore to divert substantial numbers of men and women with ill health or disability – presumably, if the medical test is working properly, those with problems that pose fewer impediments to working – into recorded unemployment, onto other benefits, or out of the benefits system altogether. 'Hidden sickness' will increase; 'recorded sickness' on disability benefits will decline.

The time-limiting of non-means tested entitlement adds to these diversions. The DWP forecast is that by 2015–16, 700,000 claimants in the Work-related Activity Group will be affected by time-limiting (DWP 2011b). The DWP also forecasts, based on information on household income, that 40 per cent (280,000) of those affected by time-limiting will not qualify for the means-tested variant of ESA. The remaining 60 per cent (420,000) will generally receive less on the means-tested variant than they did previously.

Whether those who fail to qualify for the means-tested variant of ESA will remain as a 'disability claimant' is unclear. Although they will receive no further disability benefit payment, they will remain entitled to NI credits on account of their disability, which count towards their eventual state pension entitlement. If they stay within the system in this way, they will continue to be counted as 'disabled'. On the other hand, as part of the Work-related Activity Group there will, in theory, continue to be a requirement to fulfil an 'action plan' aimed ultimately at returning to work. The experience of Jobseeker's Allowance claimants who lose entitlement to means-tested benefit is that they mostly stop their claim even though they remain unemployed, although in the case of Jobseeker's Allowance the ongoing requirements on claimants – looking for work and signing-on fortnightly – are more demanding. At least to some extent, the introduction of time-limiting seems likely to further increase the scale of 'hidden sickness' outside the benefits system.

Collectively, the reforms to disability benefits are set to have a major impact. Some 1.25 million in all can be expected to lose some or all of their financial entitlement to disability benefits – around 700,000 from time-limiting, 400,000 from re-testing and 150,000 from the refusal of new claims. The overall saving to the public purse, based on HM Treasury figures, is estimated at £4.35 billion a year by 2015–16 (Beatty and Fothergill 2013a).

*Local and regional impact*

It is perhaps to be expected that the parts of Britain with the highest disability claimant rates will be hit hardest by the reforms. In fact, in most of these places the potential reduction in disability claimant numbers and the loss of benefit income is somewhat greater than even their high claimant rate would suggest.

One reason is the geographical distribution of 'hidden unemployment'. These are the men and women claiming disability benefits who *might reasonably have been expected to be in work in a fully-employed economy* (Beatty and Fothergill 2005). Their disability claims are not fraudulent: they are men and women with ill health or disability who have accessed disability benefits rather than unemployment benefits. However, because their ill health or disability is not so severe as to prevent them from working in all circumstances, they are the group most exposed to loss of entitlement as a result of the new medical test.

'Hidden unemployed' is disproportionately concentrated in the places where the disability claimant rate is highest and the demand for labour is weakest. Where the claimant rate is low, as in large parts of southern England, the equivalent individuals have mostly been able to find work. The local impact of the disability benefit reforms can therefore be expected to be weighted towards Britain's weaker local economies. There is already evidence that this is the case. The DWP's statistics on the reassessment of existing claimants (DWP 2013: table 2) show that a higher proportion of disability claimants are being found 'fit for work' in the weaker local economies of the North of England and Wales than in the more prosperous London and South East. Only Scotland bucks the general trend, for reasons that are unclear.

The other factor skewing the local impact of disability reform is the incidence of means-testing. In London, the proportion in the Work-related Activity Group receiving only contributions-based (i.e. non-means tested) disability benefits is significantly lower than elsewhere.

Table 1

Estimated impact of disability benefit reforms by 2015–16, by region

| | No of individuals adversely affected | Estimated loss £m p.a. | No of individuals affected per 10,000 | Financial loss per working age adult £ p.a. |
|---|---|---|---|---|
| Wales | 93,000 | 320 | 480 | 165 |
| North East | 74,000 | 260 | 440 | 155 |
| North West | 197,000 | 690 | 430 | 150 |
| Scotland | 144,000 | 500 | 410 | 145 |
| Yorkshire and the Humber | 112,000 | 390 | 330 | 115 |
| West Midlands | 115,000 | 400 | 320 | 115 |
| East Midlands | 88,000 | 310 | 300 | 105 |
| South West | 92,000 | 320 | 280 | 100 |
| London | 147,000 | 470 | 260 | 85 |
| East | 83,000 | 300 | 220 | 80 |
| South East | 108,000 | 390 | 200 | 70 |
| **Great Britain** | **1,250,000** | **4,350** | **310** | **110** |

*Source:* Beatty and Fothergill 2013a, based on HM Treasury and Department for Work and Pensions data.

This indicates that fewer claimants in London risk losing their entitlement, or face a reduction in payment, when time-limiting comes into effect.

Estimates of the local and regional impact of the disability reforms, taking these factors into account, were first published when the reforms were still being introduced (Beatty and Fothergill 2011). Revised estimates of the impact (Beatty and Fothergill 2013a) are shown in tables 1 and 2. The figures here on the numbers 'adversely affected' include not only those who can be expected to lose all entitlement to disability benefits (the focus of the original 2011 estimates), but also those who can expect to have the financial value of their disability benefit reduced as means-testing comes into effect. The revised figures here also more accurately reflect the DWP's own estimates of the impact of means testing (DWP 2011b).

Table 1 shows four measures of the impact by region when the reforms have come into full effect in 2015–16. The regions are ranked here by the financial loss per adult of working age (i.e. all 16–64 year olds in the region, whether or not they claim disability benefits). This is the best measure of the intensity of the financial 'hit' facing each region. The biggest financial losses can be expected in Wales, the North East, North West and Scotland. By contrast, London, the East and South East can expect to escape relatively lightly.

Table 2

Estimated impact of disability benefit reforms by 2015–16:
worst affected 20 local authority districts in Great Britain

|  | Loss per working age adult £ p.a. |
| --- | --- |
| 1. Merthyr Tydfil | 265 |
| 2. Neath Port Talbot | 255 |
| 3. Blaenau Gwent | 255 |
| 4. Knowsley | 240 |
| 5. Rhondda Cynon Taf | 230 |
| 6. Glasgow | 225 |
| 7. Caerphilly | 225 |
| 8. Inverclyde | 220 |
| 9. Blackpool | 215 |
| 10. Barrow-in-Furness | 210 |
| 11. Liverpool | 210 |
| 12. Hartlepool | 200 |
| 13. Burnley | 200 |
| 14. Stoke-on-Trent | 200 |
| 15. West Dunbartonshire | 200 |
| 16. Barnsley | 195 |
| 17. Carmarthenshire | 195 |
| 18. Bridgend | 195 |
| 19. St Helens | 190 |
| 20. Mansfield | 190 |

*Source:* Beatty and Fothergill 2013a, based on HM Treasury
and Department for Work and Pensions data.

Table 2 shows the estimated loss, per adult of working age, in the 20
worst affected local authority districts in Britain. The three hardest hit
districts are in the Welsh Valleys, and seven of the top 20 are in South
Wales. The rest of the list (with the notable exception of Blackpool)
is a roll-call of older industrial Britain. A separate set of estimates for
Northern Ireland (Beatty and Fothergill 2013b), using essentially the
same methods, suggests that Belfast, Derry and Strabane will be hit even
harder than the worst affected districts in Great Britain.

*Impact on employment*

Ministers in the UK's coalition Government argue that the reduction in
disability benefit numbers is actually a good thing – quite apart from the
money it saves the Treasury – because married to the assistance provided
by the Work Programme it will lead to more people in employment.
They also argue that the disability reforms are best understood alongside the planned introduction of Universal Credit, which is intended

to ensure that in all circumstances claimants are financially better off in work.

What is certainly true is that for many disability claimants – the most severely ill or disabled in the Support Group are the notable exception – the reforms sharply increase the financial incentive to look for work. This is especially the case for the estimated 400,000-plus likely to lose the whole of their financial entitlement.

Labour market engagement is unquestionably set to increase. Disability claimants who are found 'fit for work' and then claim Jobseeker's Allowance instead are required to look for work. Those who retain disability benefits but are placed in the Work-related Activity Group are required to take practical steps to returning to work. These requirements are rarely likely to be popular among claimants who still perceive substantial and ongoing obstacles to working again, and it is telling that in the ten months to September 2013, almost 20,000 ESA claimants were sanctioned, three-quarters for not participating in work-related activity.

But looking for work and actually finding work are two different things. Also, if a former benefit claimant finds work this does not necessarily mean that the overall level of employment is any higher or the numbers on benefits any lower. One jobseeker can displace another in the competition to find work.

One of the ways in which extra labour supply can lead to extra employment is by addressing a shortage of labour. At various times, in various places and in particular sectors and occupations, labour shortages do unquestionably arise, but it is hard to characterize the UK in the wake of the 2008–09 recession as an economy that is especially constrained by a shortfall in labour supply. The other way in which extra labour supply can lead to extra employment is if it forces down wages so that businesses are more competitive and employers take on more workers. The problem here is that these adjustments generally take many years, and exceptionally large numbers of claimants are set to be pushed back towards the labour market over a short space of time. The adjustment is also constrained by the national minimum wage, which limits how far wages can fall.

Two further factors work against the expansion ofemployment in response to the reduction in disability benefit numbers. The first is the characteristics of the claimants themselves. Even if they are deemed 'fit for work' under the new medical test, former disability claimants will normally still be affected by health problems or disabilities that limit the work they are able to undertake. As we note above, they also tend to be an older group who previously worked mainly in low-grade manual jobs, and a high proportion have no formal qualifications. They have often been out-of-work for many years and their motivation has often been sapped. They are unlikely to be employers' first choice.

The other factor that works against an expansion of employment is the location of so many disability claimants. They are disproportionately concentrated in Britain's weakest local economies and it is the very weakest local economies of all – places such as the Welsh Valleys – that have the very highest disability claimant rates. In these places, former disability claimants face little chance of finding work.

Of course, there will be some success stories and these will no doubt be trumpeted. Some former disability claimants will find work, even perhaps in the Welsh Valleys. But to focus on individual success stories would be to miss the point. In difficult labour markets there are not enough jobs for everyone, and if one person finds a job it is most likely to be at the expense of someone else.

## Concluding Remarks

The UK's disability crisis took the best part of two decades to grow to its scale in the early 2000s and then proved largely impervious to a sustained period of economic growth and interventions by the pre-2010 Labour Government. The increase in disability claims was deeply rooted the pattern of restructuring in the UK economy and in particular in the regional and local disparities in job opportunities that arose from this restructuring. Against this backdrop, it would be rash to assume that the disability benefit numbers can easily be reduced to something closer to the low level last seen at the start of the 1980s.

There is, nevertheless, no doubt that the reforms currently underway will reduce disability claimant numbers, and there are already clear signs this is happening. Quite how far the headline numbers will fall depends on how claimants (and the employment services) react to the loss of entitlement when time-limiting takes effect. If large numbers stay on the books as 'NI credits-only' claimants, the headline numbers will fall less than if they drop out of the system altogether. Either way, the spending on disability benefits is still set to fall sharply by 2016. This will have a big impact in most of Britain's weaker local economies.

In an age of austerity, however, when jobs remain hard to find in most parts of the country, the reduction in disability numbers and spending looks set to be achieved not by moving claimants back into work but by diverting them between different parts of the benefits system or, in many cases, out of the benefits system altogether. This is hardly a lasting or satisfactory solution to the underlying problem.

It is hard to escape the conclusion, therefore, that as a tool for raising employment and economic growth the reforms to disability benefits have little value. Rather than being based upon a sound analysis of why disability claimant numbers have risen so much, and why the claimant numbers are so high in specific localities, the reforms wrongly assume that underlying problems are individuals' motivation and financial incentives, rather than ill health, disability and job opportunities. The reforms also pre-suppose that an increase in labour supply will bring forth additional labour demand, which as we explain above seems most unlikely.

As a mechanism for saving the UK Treasury substantial money, the reforms do, nevertheless, seem certain to work. Fewer people will remain entitled to disability benefits and those who retain entitlement are often likely to find that the financial value of their benefits has been reduced by means-testing. In effect, large numbers of disability claimants are being made to pay the price of a fiscal crisis that was not directly of their making. Sometimes, this financial loss will fall on households that have hitherto been able to get by tolerably well, although not necessarily very comfortably, by combining disability benefits with other sources of household income – a partner's earnings, an occupational pension, other welfare benefits. As means-testing kicks in for so many, more will be pushed down towards the poverty line. Ill health or disability, combined with unemployment, looks sets to grow as a cause of profound social and economic disadvantage.

# References

Armstrong, D. (1999), Hidden male unemployment in Northern Ireland, *Regional Studies*, 33, 6: 499–512.

Beatty, C. and Fothergill, S. (1996), Labour market adjustment in areas of chronic industrial decline: the case of the UK coalfields, *Regional Studies*, 30, 7: 637–50.

Beatty, C. and Fothergill, S. (2005), The diversion from unemployment to sickness across British regions and districts, *Regional Studies*, 39, 7: 837–54.

Beatty, C. and Fothergill, S. (2011), *Incapacity Benefit Reform: The Local, Regional and National Impact*, Sheffield: Centre for Regional Economic and Social Research, Sheffield Hallam University.

Beatty, C. and Fothergill, S. (2013a), *Hitting the Poorest Places Hardest: The Local and Regional Impact of Welfare Reform*, Sheffield: Centre for Regional Economic and Social Research, Sheffield Hallam University.

Beatty, C. and Fothergill, S. (2013b), *The Impact of Welfare Reform on Northern Ireland*, Belfast: Northern Ireland Council for Voluntary Action.

Beatty, C., Fothergill, S., Houston, D., Powell, R. and Sissons, P. (2009), *Women on Incapacity Benefits*, Sheffield: Centre for Regional Economic and Social Research, Sheffield Hallam University and University of Dundee.

Beatty, C., Fothergill, S., Houston, D., Powell, R. and Sissons, P. (2010), Bringing Incapacity Benefit numbers down: to what extent do women need a different approach? *Policy Studies*, 31, 2: 143–62.

Beatty, C., Fothergill, S. and Macmillan, R. (2000), A theory of employment, unemployment and sickness, *Regional Studies*, 34, 7: 617–30.

Bell, B. and Smith, J. (2004), *Health, Disability Insurance and Labour Force Participation*, Bank of England Working Paper No. 218, London: Bank of England.

Department for Work and Pensions (DWP) (2006), *A New Deal for Welfare: Empowering People to Work*, London: DWP.

Department for Work and Pensions (DWP) (2007), *Transformation of the Personal Capability Assessment: Technical Working Groups Phase 2 Evaluation Report*, London: DWP.

Department for Work and Pensions (DWP) (2008), *No One Written Off: Reforming Welfare to Reward Responsibility*, London: DWP.

Department for Work and Pensions (DWP) (2011a), *Press Release*, February, London: DWP.

Department for Work and Pensions (DWP) (2011b), *Impact Assessment: Time Limit Contributory Employment and Support Allowance to One Year For Those in the Work Related Activity Group*, London: DWP.

Department for Work and Pensions (DWP) (2013), *Employment and Support Allowance: Outcomes of Work Capability Assessments, Great Britain*, Quarterly Official Statistics Bulletin, April 2013, London: DWP.

Fieldhouse, E. and Hollywood, E. (1999), Life after mining; hidden unemployment and changing patterns of economic activity among miners in England and Wales 1981–91, *Work, Employment and Society*, 13, 3: 483–502.

HM Treasury (2013), *Budget 2013*, London: HM Treasury.

Kemp, P. (2006), Comparing trends in disability benefit receipt. In P. Kemp, A. Sunden and B. Bakker Tauritz (eds), *Sick Societies? Trends in Disability Benefits in Post-Industrial Welfare States*, Geneva: International Social Security Association.

Kemp, P. A. and Davidson, J. (2010), Employability trajectories among new claimants of Incapacity Benefit, *Policy Studies*, 31, 2: 203–21.

Lindsay, C. and Houston, D. (2013), *Disability Benefits, Welfare Reform and Employment Policy*, Basingstoke: Palgrave Macmillan.

Little, A. (2007), Inactivity and labour market attachment in Britain, *Scottish Journal of Political Economy*, 54, 1: 19–52.

MacKay, R. (1999), Work and nonwork: a more difficult labour market, *Environment and Planning A*, 31, 11: 919–34.

McVicar, D. (2006), Why do disability benefit rolls vary between regions? A review of evidence from the US and UK, *Regional Studies*, 40, 5: 519–33.

McVicar, D. (2008), Why have UK disability rolls grown so much? *Journal of Economic Surveys*, 22, 1: 114–39.

McVicar, D. (2013), Local level incapacity benefit claimant rolls in Britain: correlates and convergence, *Regional Studies*, 47, 8: 1267–82.

National Audit Office (2010), *Support to Incapacity Benefits Claimants through Pathways to Work*, London: Stationery Office.

Webster, D. (2002), Unemployment: how official statistics distort analysis and policy, and why, *Radical Statistics*, 79/80: 96–127.

Webster, D. (2004), *Sickness, Invalidity and Incapacity Benefit Claimants over 6 months 1963–2004, based on calculations using Social Security Statistics*, personal communication.

Webster, D., Arnott, J., Brown, J., Turok, I., Mitchell, R. and Macdonald, E. (2010), Falling Incapacity Benefit claims in a former industrial city: policy impacts or labour market improvement? *Policy Studies*, 31, 2: 163–85.

Webster, D., Brown, J., Macdonald, E. and Turok, I. (2013), The interaction of health, labour market conditions and long-term sickness benefit claims in a post-industrial city: a Glasgow case study. In C. Lindsay and D. Houston (eds), *Disability Benefits, Welfare Reform and Employment Policy*, Basingstoke: Palgrave Macmillan, pp. 111–33.

# 3

# From Impairment to Incapacity – Educational Inequalities in Disabled People's Ability to Work

## Ben Baumberg

## Introduction

Prior to the financial crisis, 6 per cent of the working-age population in countries of the Organisation for Economic Co-operation and Development (OECD) were claiming disability-related benefits (OECD 2010: 59). While more recent figures on benefits claims are hard to come by, in 2013 there were still more working-age (15–64) people inactive due to illness, disability or retirement across the EU than the number who were unemployed.[1] The distinction between unemployment and disability-related benefits is important because incapacitated people – i.e. those who are unable to work due to sickness or disability – are widely felt to deserve special treatment (van Oorschot 2006). As a result, incapacity benefits predate unemployment benefits (Kangas 2010), and while there has been an increasing activation of incapacity claimants, they still generally receive higher benefit levels with fewer attached conditions.

The most common interpretation is that these high incapacity claim levels do *not* reflect genuinely high levels of an inability to work. Instead, bodies such as the OECD (2003: 169) argue that there has been a 'policy failure' that encourages people to *choose* to claim incapacity benefits. Partly, this reflects an economic model of rational decision-making, given evidence that claimant rates are influenced by incentives (McVicar 2006) – sometimes with the implication that claimants are 'malingering'. But more influential has been the biopsychosocial model (Wade and Halligan 2004), according to which the policy failure has been allowing people to believe that they are incapable of work and to become 'dependent' on benefits.

This view has been contested by those who focus on how weak labour demand constrains choice. Beatty and Fothergill have influentially

*New Perspectives on Health, Disability, Welfare and the Labour Market*, First Edition.
Edited by Colin Lindsay, Bent Greve, Ignazio Cabras, Nick Ellison and Stephen Kellett.
© 2015 John Wiley & Sons, Ltd. Published 2015 by John Wiley & Sons, Ltd.

described incapacity claimants as the 'hidden unemployed' (Beatty *et al.* 2000), amid extensive evidence that plant closures lead to rises in inca- pacity receipt, and that incapacity claimants are primarily low-skilled people in areas with few jobs (Houston and Lindsay 2010; Beatty *et al.* 2009). This is not to suggest that claimants are non-disabled; Beatty and Fothergill recognize that disability may be a factor in losing work and being left at the back of the 'queue for jobs' (Beatty *et al.* 2009). Funda- mentally, though, disability is a criteria for sorting the unemployed, and the 'hidden unemployed' are not seen as incapacitated.

This account is in many ways compelling (Houston and Lindsay 2010), yet it does not consider whether inequalities in benefit receipt may partly be due to *genuine* incapacity; indeed, it is striking that neither the biopsychosocial or hidden unemployment models consider incapac- ity in any depth. Beatty and Fothergill (2005) ignore health inequalities, despite evidence that mortality explains at least as much of the spatial variation in incapacity claims as labour demand (McVicar 2009). More- over, 'incapacity' means that work risks the health of the worker; or risks the health of others; or – crucially – that the person is unable to work to the expected level (Palmer and Cox 2007). It is therefore possible that incapacity – beyond ill-health *per se* – is more common among disadvan- taged people in disadvantaged places.

This article therefore presents the results of a qualitative study that investigated the differential ability of people with different educational levels to avoid incapacity in the face of an impairment. The article starts by reviewing evidence on work and incapacity, before presenting the methods and results, and concluding with the implications for research and policy.

## Literature review

To understand the limits of the hidden unemployment approach, we need to use the social model of disability, where 'disability' is not an inherent property of an individual but the result of individual functional impairments combined with a disabling social environment (Barnes 2000).[2] Incapacity (work disability) therefore cannot be a binary, med- ical determination; as the London School of Economics (LSE) founder and social activist Sidney Webb put it in 1914, 'incapable of any work whatsoever' can only mean 'literally unconscious or asleep' (cited by Gulland 2011: 7). Incapacity therefore fundamentally depends upon the nature of work – and while it also depends upon people's beliefs and local labour demand, these three factors tend to be separated into three distinct literatures.

Still, there is an extensive quantitative literature that links working conditions to incapacity. One of the most influential models is Ilmari- nen's 'work ability house' (Maltby 2011), which primarily considers health, professional competence, values and the nature of work. There is good evidence that work-related factors influence the most common measure of work ability (van den Berg *et al.* 2009), but this only offers a blurred measure of incapacity as it includes direct measures of health. This reflects a general problem with the wider quantitative literature, including studies using the demands-control model (Baumberg 2014), which generally do not enable us to tease apart whether working conditions impact on ill-health *per se* versus whether working conditions make it harder for a person with a given level of ill-health to work. This is a crucial distinction, given that health does not explain the observed socio-economic inequalities in incapacity receipt (Østby *et al.* 2011).

Qualitative research is potentially more promising in separating these two explanations, given that it can trace the complex processes through which factors have causal effects (Maxwell 2004). Studies of incapacity nearly always thickly describe the incapacitating effect of the pace and intensity of work, and also the ways in which employer adjustments and phased returns-to-work can avoid incapacity (e.g. Gewurtz and Kirs 2009; Sainsbury *et al.* 2008: 64). Yet many of the medically-oriented studies simply list the factors that mattered within that particular sample (e.g. Kennedy *et al.* 2007; Liedberg and Henriksson 2002), rather than constructing a theoretical account of how these factors *in combination* limit the possibilities available for different people. And while they sometimes consider biopsychosocial factors, they rarely offer any integration with Beatty's and Fothergill's account of hidden unemployment.

The gaps in knowledge can perhaps be most clearly seen when looking at two of the most nuanced accounts. Johansson's illness flexibility model (Johansson and Lundberg 2004; Hansson *et al.* 2006) considers how 'requirements' (constraints), 'incentives' and job flexibility (see below) influence sickness absence. Likewise, longitudinal qualitative research by the Social Policy Research Unit at the University of York (Sainsbury and Davidson 2006; Irvine 2011; Sainsbury *et al.* 2008) captures the unfolding influence of nearly every known factor on employment among disabled people. Yet in their desire to capture multiple influences, neither study fully explores people's *ability* to work, nor whether lower-skilled people with an impairment have fewer abilities to work – leaving us with a critical gap in this valuable comprehensive literature. To our knowledge, the present study is the first to combine these disparate literatures and focus specifically on whether there are educational inequalities in how impairment becomes incapacity.

## Methodology

Rather than aiming to be statistically representative, this sample aimed to cover the range of variation within the wider population (Ritchie and Lewis 2003), focusing on:

1. type of health condition;
2. whether the person left work;
3. gender; and
4. education level.

Table 1

Properties of the main sample

| | |
|---|---|
| Age 20s/30s | 12 |
| Age 40s | 13 |
| Age 50+ | 7 |
| No qualifications | 6 |
| NVQ Level 1 qualifications | 3 |
| NVQ Level 2 qualifications | 8 |
| NVQ Level 3 qualifications | 6 |
| Degree-level qualifications | 8 |
| Male | 16 |
| Female | 16 |
| Mental health condition | 13 |
| Physical health condition | 19 |
| Has claimed incapacity benefits (IB/ESA) | 14 |
| Not claimed incapacity benefits | 18 |
| Left work due to health problem | 18 |
| Stayed in work | 14 |

*Notes:* IB = Incapacity Benefit; ESA = Employment and Support Allowance.

Participants were purposively recruited through five general practitioner (GP) practices across advantaged and disadvantaged areas, within which waiting patients were invited to take part. Volunteers were then screened by phone, selecting only working-age individuals who had recently had a health problem that interfered with their work, and achieving balance according to the criteria above. In total, 341 people were approached, of whom 139 were successfully screened, 41 passed, and 28 interviews were conducted (October 2009 to June 2010). While the sample was varied in most respects, it became clear that it contained relatively few incapacity claimants, and 11 further claimants were obtained through three offices of a Welfare-to-Work provider.

A target of around 35–45 interviews was expected to be sufficient to obtain sufficient variation (Manderbacka 1998: 320), but this 'saturation' was actually reached at a slightly earlier point, and the analyses below are based on 32 interviews.[3] This resulted in a sample that was varied in all key respects (see table 1); and also by type of work (see table S1).

The interviews focused on the extent to which impairments led to problems with fitness-for-work in a previous job and the options that people then had available, based on respondents' descriptions of their impairments (see below). In-depth interviews were chosen to investigate individual narratives and minimize social influence effects, using a topic guide developed through two pilot interviews. Participants were given a choice of interview location; most were at home but some were conducted in cafes/pubs, and several were conducted in a private room at the Welfare-to-Work provider. The research received ethical approval from the LSE Ethics Committee, the National Health Service Research Ethics Service (reference 08/H0714/110), and the Research Management team within each primary care trust.

The interviews lasted 35–135 minutes, and after transcription were analyzed using a combination of thematic coding and the Framework method (Ritchie and Lewis 2003). This meant that a draft coding frame was developed based on previous literature and an initial subsample. Each transcript was then read two to three times and coded in NVivo, before being summarized in a charting framework that covered key themes. The final analysis used both the framework (to compare cases) and the codes (to compare themes and extract quotes) to build a theoretical model linking impairment to incapacity, before examining the role of education and wider socioeconomic factors in these pathways.

## Results

From the outset, it was clear that people faced different levels of choices in responding to impairments, and that these partly reflected their educational level. This is vividly illustrated when we compare Lindsey (with GCSEs) to Maryah (with a degree).

Lindsey had managed her depression for many years while working in charity shops, but had been finding it increasingly difficult to cope. She said that everyone thought her assistant manager job *'was a doddle'*, but it was actually *'very pressurised'* given the weekly targets from management – and trying to speak to the employer about the workload was simply seen as *'making excuses'*. This left a *'vicious circle'* of pressure and depression, where she was isolating herself from friends and family. When her otherwise understanding manager took out a bad day on her, she thought, *'I just thought "no, I can't deal with this anymore", and I just … put my notice in'* – although if it had not been for this argument, she felt she could not have carried on much longer.

This was during the recession, and Lindsey soon realized it was a bad time to be looking for work – the *'dole queues will be flooded with people'* looking for retail work. Yet applying for benefits would simply have been swapping the pressure of her old job for the pressure of the Jobcentre, so she instead got by on the little savings she had. Ten months after leaving her job her savings had run out and she *'couldn't see any hope'*, so she took an overdose. Her sister came as soon as she received the suicide note, took her to hospital, and later filled in the benefit application forms. By the time she participated in this study she was somewhat better and thinking about returning to work. Employment in a supermarket seemed unlikely (an occupational health assessor had concerns about her ability to cope), but she had been doing a small amount of permitted work in a dry cleaners, who she felt were unusually understanding.

Maryah also suffered from *'stress'*, but in nearly every other way her experiences were different. She was a marketing director for a global cosmetics firm in a job she described as *'un-doable'*, being responsible for 16 countries across Europe, which she juggled with being a single mother. While loving the challenge, in the last six months of this job she began to struggle, *'I was waking up every morning at 4 o'clock, just bad dreams, being on fire alive or jumping off a high tower or whatever. It was clearly stress-related'*. When her child therapist said her daughter's problems were related to her stress, she decided to change job. She felt that reducing the stress of her existing job was impossible – *'if [a boss] sees that you have been doing the job for a year without an extra assistant or manager, why get one?'* – but instead told her boss that she *'wants out'*. She moved to a less-stressful job with the same company, but this was less satisfying and she ultimately negotiated a leaving package before having another child with a new partner. At the time of our interview she was looking to work again but was avoiding stressful jobs after the 'permanent damage' inflicted by her old job. With her contacts, money and skills she was thinking of various types of self-employment, some of which thought would be 'really easy' to achieve.

While there are obvious similarities in these two stories – they are both people dealing with stress at work, albeit of different kinds – the options available to them were very different. But how can we understand these differences? To theorize what is happening more systematically, we need to break apart this complexity into several different responses to workplace impairments, of which there seemed to be three that span the diversity of the previous literatures: flexibility, employer adjustments and changing job.

## Using flexibility

The quickest and most straightforward response to a fitness-for-work limitation was for workers to change their work themselves to fit around it, if they had sufficient autonomy (Sainsbury *et al.* 2008: 134). Workplace autonomy is a complex concept (Hodgson 2004): irrespective of people's meaningful levels of control over their work, what was crucial here was whether people had the right sort of flexibility for their impairments. For example, Cheryl's office job enabled her to get up and stretch her back whenever she wanted – something that was simply not available to Khaled as a bus driver, causing him considerable pain (see below).

One form of flexibility that was particularly important was what Johansson and Lundberg (2004: 1859) call 'adjustment latitude': 'the opportunity people have to reduce or in other ways alter their work effort when e.g. feeling ill' (see also Gewurtz and Kirs 2009: 40). This enabled people with fluctuating conditions to alter the order or pace of their work to reflect their moment-to-moment abilities, as Yvette explained for her auditing job:

> ' "Do I work as quickly when I'm in a lot of pain?" I think well hand on heart I've got to say no [...] You know, the amount of work I do at the end of the day is the same, but it takes more effort and, you know, if I feel like one day I've had a crap day, then maybe the next day I'll try and work harder.'

At extremes, workers could pretend to work rather than taking sickness absence, even on days when they were unable to do any work at all, *'I said I was going looking for properties [...] and I'd come home and I'd just lie down all day, and not get a sick note'* (Nick, property finance). Without adjustment latitude, impaired performance was more visible to employers. Sarah worked 'incredibly hard' as a supermarket supervisor on some days, but had other days where her depression made her unable to work productively. That she managed to stay in her job so long was not because she had the adjustment latitude to conceal this, but rather because of her previous manager:

> *'I remember my direct manager saying to me one time, "You know what? You're the best supervisor I've ever had. Because even though you've got your illness, some days you get really unmotivated and you can't actually do anything [...] But on the days that you're on the ball, you try so hard." [...] And if it weren't for that man, my direct manager, I don't think I would've survived the last eight years [...] If it weren't for [him] protecting me and backing me up, [the management] would've gone full-pelt at me because there's been many times they tried to get me sacked.'*

As this suggests, flexibility was not available to everyone. Khaled's bus driving was inflexible, partly governed by passengers and partly by managerial surveillance (motion sensors, cameras). While the present study focused on processes of incapacity rather than of work design, adjustment latitude appeared to be an integral feature of jobs where managerial control was exercised through targets or the allocation of discrete packages of work. We have already seen how Nick had very high levels of adjustment latitude that enabled him to avoid sickness absence, and elsewhere he described his job as follows, *'If you want to take longer for lunch, take longer for lunch. If you want to turn up late, turn up late. But you're going to have to do the work somewhere along the way, it's up to you when you do it'.*

But what of the link between education and autonomy? The qualitative design of the present study does not enable us to make robust generalizations based on patterns of association, much as lower-educated respondents like Khaled and Sarah tended to have less flexibility, while higher-educated respondents like Nick and Yvette had more flexibility.

There are also many influences on autonomy for any given job in any given workplace, ranging from the structural to the individual manager. Still, it is clear from other, quantitative research that forms of autonomy tend to cluster together, and that autonomy is strongly socially patterned (Baumberg 2011); indeed, autonomy is part of the *definition* of NS-SEC (National Statistics Socioeconomic classification) social classes. Flexibility can help prevent impairments turning into incapacity, and as we return to below, it is more likely to be available for some people than others.

## Employer adjustments

At times, flexibility could be replaced by employer adjustments. In particular, for people who struggled to maintain a fixed posture for long periods, employers could allow more frequent breaks to reduce pain and physical strain. Hence while Cheryl (above) had the flexibility to take breaks within her job, Helen was granted permission by her employer to get up from her desk and stretch her back regularly.

Yet the importance of employer adjustments went far beyond this (Sainsbury *et al.* 2008: 157). A lot of people's physical impairments were *task-specific* – that is, they struggled with a specific aspect of the job, such as holding fixed postures, lifting heavy objects, bending, etc. Employers could therefore make adjustments to either modify the physical environment (e.g. Nick received a phone headset to reduce neck pain), or to remove the specific disabling aspects of people's jobs. Adjustments could be formal or informal, and could also occur for people with mental health difficulties: cleaning the shopping centre on busy, rainy dates was too chaotic for Yusuf to deal with given his post-traumatic stress disorder, so on these days he was sent to clean empty stairwells instead.

These adjustments helped people stay in work, but again they were not available for everyone. One disadvantage of adjustments *vis-à-vis* flexibility is that people had to disclose their impairment to their employer, and some people were unwilling to do this for fear of losing the job. Khaled would have benefited from being allowed regular breaks to stretch his back, as we have already seen for Helen and Cheryl. However, he said that, *'I'd rather not [tell them about my disability] because … I don't feel that they would appreciate the fact that I have back problem […] Anything under five years [working there] they can get rid of you easily'.* Nor would adjustments occur where they involved tasks that were central to the job, such as Tessa's epilepsy making it hard for her to care for children.

Adjustments were valuable where they were possible, where an employee was confident enough to request them, and where an employer was happy to grant them. Small adjustments around desk-based work were sometimes possible for people in office jobs with little flexibility, and more significant adjustments were sometimes possible for people with physical impairments in physical jobs – and these people were *not* necessarily highly-educated.

*Adjusting demands*

Another type of adjustment was a phased return to work, where work-load was temporarily reduced after absence (Gewurtz and Kirs 2009; Sainsbury *et al.* 2008: 64) – an adjustment that can be thought of as responding to temporary 'sickness' rather than (semi-)permanent 'disability'. This was important for many impairments relating to the pace/intensity of work, which could be physical (e.g. standing/sitting for long periods) or stress-related. Yet there seemed to participants almost no scope whatsoever for *permanently* reducing demands, other than reducing the hours of work (see below). Marjorie would have been able to do her cleaning work without bending down if she could reduce her work pace, but instead had to give up the job. Scott put it similarly, *'There is no room for manoeuvre. I know as far as I was concerned, the pressure was always going to be there if I went back to that job'*. Others tried and failed to persuade their employers to reduce their demands, and as shown for Lindsey and Maryah above, this applied irrespective of their education. People also sometimes felt that their mental health made it difficult to deal with demands that other people could cope with, *'I'm not [my man-ager]. I'm me. It's what I can reasonably do. What my strength is suited for. But they don't see it like that'* (Lindsey). Indeed, employees with impairments may actually find themselves with a higher workload than others, to the extent that their impairment makes it more difficult to resist excessive workload demands. As Sarah put it, other supermarket staff would say, *'just don't pressure me'* to managers, but *'I can't do that, I'd end up bursting into tears'*.

In the face of a near-universal inability to permanently reduce demands, perhaps the most revealing situation was that of Ricardo. He had been in bed for ten months after a serious motorbike accident, and when his health started to improve, he found a job through a friend as a caretaker at a church. This job was perfect for his situation, with a low and flexible pace of work – he reported that his boss said, *'I don't care about the time, there's room for five months, I don't care. Just do it nicely. [...] If you don't come tomorrow don't worry about it, just take your time and do your work you can'*. Uniquely here, this situation was allowed to continue indefinitely. Tellingly, Ricardo described this job as *'a gesture'*. By this he implied that it was an act of charity by a religious organization, which in its exceptional nature highlights the impossibility of permanently reduc-ing demands within the normal logic of work.

*Changing job*

The final way to make impairments less-disabling was to move to a more suitable job – a major feature of people's accounts, but surprisingly rarely studied in the wider literature, even in the 'hidden unemploy-ment' literature that it most closely relates to.

Almost by definition, more 'employable' people found it easier to move. (While we use 'employability' to refer to an individual's ability to find work, this is obviously specific to particular labour markets at particular times [see McQuaid and Lindsay 2005].) Employability was partly a matter of qualifications, but also reflected age and language skills and a general difficulty in finding work in late 2009/early 2010. Even those with some relevant skills/experience were sometimes concerned, with Cheryl having experience and a childcare diploma but still feeling that childcare work is *'difficult because there's lots of mums that want it'*. This is also described by Beatty and Fothergill, where the 'hidden unemployed' are formed of those with genuine impairments who find themselves out of work at times and places where there is a shortage of jobs.

But there is more to it than this. When people were moving jobs, they were not just trying to get *any* job, they were trying to get a *suitable* job, one that did not conflict with their particular impairment – and this does not feature in Beatty's and Fothergill's account. Often this meant changing career entirely, to fields that did not match their experience or qualifications, and even higher-educated respondents could find this challenging. Elizabeth and Naveed both felt that changing careers in their 40s (from nursing and martial arts instruction, respectively) would be hard. Nevertheless, while Naveed was worried – *'what other skills have I got to offer that would attract employers apart from the fact that I'm a graduate?'* – he was still considering retraining in social work if necessary.

Better-qualified people may have been reluctant to change career, but the greatest difficulties were for those with lower qualifications. Damian was a case in point. His depression made him unable to concentrate sufficiently to continue working as an electrician, *'I nearly killed a bunch of work mates just by not concentrating on my wiring of things'*. While it would have been easy to continue as an electrician – he had friends working in the trade who kept offering him work – the wooziness from his medication made this impossible. With no relevant experience or qualifications he was therefore looking for 'menial jobs', and *'like a mug [I was] thinking I'm going to walk straight back into another job [...] It was like everyone says, it's not that easy at the moment'*. This left him in a 'Catch-22' situation where he was not employable enough to get the jobs he was fit to do, and not fit enough to do the jobs he could get.

Ali also fell into this Catch-22. His previous work as a chef in an Indian restaurant was now too physically demanding, and he had to try and find a job despite his poor English language skills and lack of qualifications, *'If I got a good education, then I got a choice, I can do [chef work] or not, take it or leave it. Because I haven't got any education. I have to do it'*. He was therefore resigned to claiming incapacity benefits, until whichever among death and retirement came first. Similar binds also applied to some lower-qualified workers who were struggling and unable to change to a more suitable job, as we explore further below.

Yet it is not as simple as saying that all higher-educated people could find suitable work while lower-educated people could not. Irrespective of people's level of education, if their impairment still allowed them to do work that used some of their previous skills, then it was easier to find suitable work. This applied to several people who wanted to do less stressful versions of their previous jobs, such as Scott and Steve who expected to find voluntary-sector information technology roles at a much lower level of intensity. In contrast, better-educated people in the sample with more severe disabilities were still unlikely to find suitable work. Disability discrimination was also widely-reported, with many reporting that no one would employ them if they revealed their disability.

Finding suitable work also had an element of chance. Redeployment, for example, was only possible in certain large employers such as the police force; Helen said that otherwise, *'I'd be out of work. I don't think anyone would employ me with my medical history'*. Perhaps the luckiest people, though, were where someone else found them an unusually understanding employer. Ricardo's exceptional caretaking job (above) was found for him through a church friend; Yusuf's sympathetic cleaning job by his welfare-to-work provider; and it was Cheryl's mother who found her a job that eased her back to work gently, working only until lunchtime until she felt capable of doing more:

> *'[The job] fell in my lap really. I didn't actively go out, my mum phoned me one day and she said "We need some temps" [ . . . ] . . . when I had to go home, and I had to go home because I was just getting in a state, it was, "Fine, go on, off you go." [...] I'm thankful for that because I don't know how I would get back into employment otherwise'*

Cheryl, Yusuf, Ricardo and Helen all recognized their good fortune in finding suitable jobs. Without this, they all expected to face the Catch-22 of not being employable enough to get the jobs they were fit to do, and not fit enough to do the jobs they could get.

### Choice and constraint

The analysis in this article suggests that some people with impairments were able to find non-disabling work environments, through job flexibility, job adjustments, or moving to a more suitable job. However, this did not result in a black-and-white situation where people were either fully fit-for-work or fully incapacitated. Instead, there was a sizeable grey area where people were 'struggling on' (Sainsbury and Davidson 2006) with impairments that partially interfered with their job. This introduces the possibility of further inequalities in the extent to which people are allowed to – and feel compelled to – struggle on.

Some inequalities were around whether employers would accept sickness absence and/or reduced performance. While this varied from manager to manager, employers generally seemed sympathetic for temporary sickness (such as an operation), but less so for chronic disability (long-term or repeated short-term absences). Melanie was not alone in feeling pressures to minimize absence, *'You're just forever getting warnings whenever you're sick… When an ambulance is called to work [after going into a diabetic coma], I won't let them take me away because that will by my percentage [that monitors absence] gone up again … So it's not a good place to be'.*

Moreover, sickness absence policies were a way dealing with poor performance. No one (at least in this sample, but see Sainsbury *et al.* 2008) was sacked directly on performance grounds, but poor performance instead could be *transformed into* a problem of absence by applying continual pressure. For example, Sarah suspected that pressure – which she experienced as 'bullying' – was being deliberately applied to her in order for her to take sickness absence, a tactic that was ultimately successful.

Some struggling workers therefore had decisions taken out of their hands. The remainder had to decide whether to accept the physical and psychological burden of struggling (Wilton 2008). Continuing to work sometimes damaged their health or put them in considerable pain, and the effort of staying in work often came to dominate their lives. As Erica put it, talking about her job with a major budget clothing retailer with a workload she described as *'mental'*, *'I'm not physically capable of this 20 hours a week, running this house – which isn't a lot because you can see the state of it (laughs) – and a private life. I'm not capable of it all and I just literally don't have a private life. No friends, no boyfriend – no nothing'.*

Given that it was almost unheard of for employers to permanently reduce job demands, the main options left were to reduce hours, change job, or leave work. Crucially, though, individuals not employers bore this cost, and this was only a 'choice' if people could cope with reduced income. Khaled was one of those who felt financially trapped. He was forced to sit down for nine hours in his job as a bus driver, leading to back pain he described as *'like having a knife in your back, cutting across'*, and he was too exhausted when he got home to socialize, even after ceasing overtime. Khaled felt he could have claimed incapacity benefits (his injury was visible on MRI scans), or changed to a retail job (with his cousin) – but both of these would lead to what he considered to be an unacceptable drop in income, forcing him to deny his kids the right *'to have that just* little bit *extra'*. While this may sound like a 'choice', it certainly wasn't experienced as such – *'It's recommended [by doctors] to do something else, but (…) there's not much that can be done'.*

In other words, some people not only had more options available to find non-disabling work (above), but when they had partial fitness-for-work limitations, they also had more choice about whether to struggle on.

## Discussion

In reflecting on these findings, it is important to be mindful of the study's limitations. This method does not aim for a survey's 'representational generalization'; instead it aims for 'theoretical generalization' based on a sample that contains variety in the phenomenon of interest (Ritchie and Lewis 2003). This is subject to several caveats: that some less common experiences have been missed (e.g. bipolar disorder), as will those who avoid formal services (GPs, welfare-to-work providers), and the interviews were limited to London. Furthermore, the interview data was treated as a valid account of people's experiences, and while we make our own judgements as to the degree that people were incapacitated, this builds from people's own accounts of how their impairments affected their lives. Interviews will also be affected both by the author's own particular social position and the embedding of such interviews within participants' wider narratives.

A further issue – rarely addressed explicitly – concerns causal inference in qualitative research. The analysis here focused on 'process tracing': that is, examining the unfolding sequences of events within each person, looking for evidence of which complex constellation of factors leads to the observed outcomes, comparing all the cases to one another and paying particular attention to exceptions (Maxwell 2004). No method of causal inference is infallible, however. Furthermore, while we trace the processes through which impairment becomes incapacity, some of these processes are only indirectly related to education. For these we draw on wider evidence, and suggest further avenues for research below. With these limitations in mind, this discussion summarizes the article's results in the context of the wider literature, and draws out the implications for research and policy.

## Findings

Based on an in-depth analysis of interviews with 32 individuals with physical and mental impairments, this article suggests that some people have systematic advantages in preventing their impairments from becoming incapacitating, going beyond the existing literatures on hidden unemployment and working conditions. More precisely, it suggests that both workplace inequalities and labour market inequalities are at work:

- Job flexibility enabled people to work around their impairment, as found in both qualitative (Sainsbury *et al.* 2008: 134; Gewurtz and Kirs 2009: 40) and quantitative research (Allebeck and Mastekaasa 2004: 57; Baumberg 2014). Such flexibility was more common among better-educated people – but the present, qualitative study cannot offer robust evidence of such patterns of association. However, nationally representative surveys of work confirm that high-autonomy jobs tend to be more common among better-educated people (Baumberg 2011).
- Changing to a more suitable job also enabled people to find non-disabling work environments, for which better qualifications directly helped. This goes beyond the important Beatty and Fothergill account: it is not (just) that less employable people found it harder to find work ('hidden unemployment'), but that they found it harder to find *suitable* work, which meant they were *genuinely* incapacitated.

Some low-qualified people who had to move field therefore faced a Catch-22 situation where they were not employable enough to get the jobs that their health allowed them to do, but not fit enough to do the jobs that they were skilled or experienced enough to get – leaving only a remote possibility of finding suitable work.

This is not to suggest that all lower-qualified people had no options. They too were sometimes able to move into more suitable jobs through a fortuitous combination of events, or could be in the sorts of jobs where employer adjustments could make a difference. Yet while it is a legal obligation in many countries to make 'reasonable' adjustments, the bar of 'reasonableness' is high – some tasks are too important to be removed; studies of employers found they are worried about the resentment they induce among colleagues (Sainsbury *et al.* 2008: 89); and permanent reductions in workload are rare (as also found in Gewurtz and Kirs 2009; Sainsbury *et al.* 2008: 91–2). While education did not determine outcomes on its own, there were simply fewer ways of avoiding incapacity among lower-educated respondents.

Beyond this, there is a further dimension of inequality around whether people had control over 'struggling on' (Sainsbury and Davidson 2006) in a partly-disabling environment. Employers sometimes pressurized struggling workers to take sickness absence, and then terminated the contracts of workers with long-term absence or repeated short-term absence (Sainsbury and Davidson 2006: 38–51). Furthermore, people themselves questioned whether they wanted to continue struggling in the face of pain and exhaustion (Wilton 2008). Reduced hours were a common response, yet it is notable that the costs of this are borne by the worker themselves. The viability of both reduced hours and stopping work therefore depended on their ability to cope with reduced income, and again, there is extensive evidence that income/wealth are associated with education (Karagiannaki 2011).

It is worth clarifying the basis on which these conclusions have been made. The study itself showed the processes through which certain people had choices in responding to impairments, whereas others had none. Education's role in increasing the choices available was partly direct (for employability), but partly a matter of indirect probabilistic relationships (for flexibility and wealth) confirmed in other studies. While further research is necessary (see below), it is clear that incapacity results from the *combination* of impairments with disabling work environments, and it seems that better-educated people were better able to stop impairments becoming incapacitating – a finding whose implications we now consider for both research and policy.

## Implications

A first implication relates to academic debates. This study suggests that the concentration of incapacity claims in lower-qualified people may not just be a matter of 'hidden unemployment' as Beatty and Fothergill suggest, but because lower-qualified people are genuinely more incapacitated, due to workplace factors and their interactions with labour market factors. However, while the processes underlying hidden unemployment are extensively documented, the processes underlying incapacity are less so. De Raeve *et al.* (2009) found people were more likely to change jobs after becoming psychologically distressed; Gignac *et al.* (2008) found that 21 per cent of people with arthritis changed jobs; and Jones and Latreille (2011) found that disabled people were more likely to become self-employed – but otherwise there are surprisingly few studies focused on occupational change as a response to impairments. Moreover, while we know that highly-educated disabled people suffer a pay penalty compared to non-disabled people (Longhi *et al.* 2009), it is unclear if this penalty extends to other factors such as adjustment latitude. Further research is necessary, including quantitative research that looks directly at the respective prevalence of job flexibility, adjustments and occupational change among people with impairments, and how this varies across people of different educational levels in different local labour markets.

The findings also directly relate to debates around how we should assess incapacity within the benefits system. If incapacity by definition depends on labour market disadvantage as well as impairment, then there is a strong case for considering such factors when assessing incapacity. This has been done, for example, in Sweden up until the late 1990s (Kemp *et al.* 2006) and there have been calls to introduce such a 'real-world' assessment in the UK (Citizens Advice Bureau 2010). However, the Government's independent reviewer of the incapacity assessment recently dismissed this policy because we 'lacked the necessary detail and evidence base' (Harrington 2011: 37). Furthermore, while space precludes a full discussion (see Baumberg 2011; Baumberg 2014), it may be possible to reduce incapacity by both better-matching people with impairments to suitable jobs, and by making workplaces generally less disabling.

If further study confirms and extends the findings here, then there is therefore the possibility of creating a fairer system of incapacity assessment, and of reducing the rate of incapacity *per se*. On these grounds, inequalities in responses to impairments would seem worth exploring in future research.

## Acknowledgements

Thanks to two anonymous reviewers, Annie Irvine (and others at SPRU) and John Hills (and others at CASE) for their help – which does not indicate their agreement with the views here. Thanks also to the Welfare-to-Work provider and GP surgeries who facilitated this study, and especially to the people who spoke to me about their lives.

## Notes

1. LFS figures for 2013, http://ec.europa.eu/eurostat/web/lfs/data/database (accessed 23 May 2014).
2. 'Impairment' here refers to an inability to perform specific tasks, while 'disability' refers to the inability to perform a given social role. This follows analogous distinctions in, for example, the World Health Organization's *International Classification of Functioning, Disability and Health*, http://www.who.int/classifications/icf/en/ (accessed 23 May 2014).
3. After analyzing 24 transcripts, it became clear that saturation was being reached for some types of claimant; eight further interviews were therefore purposively selected for analysis.

## References

Allebeck, P. and Mastekaasa, A. (2004), Chapter 5. Risk factors for sick leave – general studies, *Scandinavian Journal of Public Health*, 32: 49–108.

Barnes, C. (2000), A working social model? Disability, work and disability politics in the 21st century, *Critical Social Policy*, 20, 4: 441–57.

Baumberg, B. (2011), *The role of increasing job strain in deteriorating fitness-for-work and rising incapacity benefit receipt*, PhD thesis, London: The London School of Economics and Political Science.

Baumberg, B. (2014), Fit-for-work – or work fit for disabled people? The role of changing job demands and control in incapacity Claims, *Journal of Social Policy*, 43: 289–310.

Beatty, C. and Fothergill, S. (2005), The diversion from 'unemployment' to 'sickness' across British regions and districts, *Regional Studies*, 39, 7: 837–54.

Beatty, C., Fothergill, S. and Macmillan, R. (2000), A theory of employment, unemployment and sickness, *Regional Studies*, 34, 7: 617–30.

Beatty, C., Fothergill, S., Houston, D., Powell, R. and Sissons, P. (2009), A gendered theory of employment, unemployment and sickness, *Environment and Planning C: Government and Policy*, 27, 6: 958–74.

Citizens Advice Bureau (2010), *Not Working: CAB Evidence on the ESA Work Capability Assessment*, London: Citizens Advice Bureau.

De Raeve, L., Kant, I., Jansen, N. W. H., Vasse, R. M. and van den Brandt, P. A. (2009), Changes in mental health as a predictor of changes in working time arrangements and occupational mobility: results from a prospective cohort study, *Journal of Psychosomatic Research*, 66, 2: 137–45.

Gewurtz, R. and Kirs, B. (2009), Disruption, disbelief and resistance: a meta-synthesis of disability in the workplace, *Work*, 34, 1: 33–44.

Gignac, M. A. M., Cao, X., Lacaille, D., Anis, A. H. and Badley, E. M. (2008), Arthritis-related work transitions: a prospective analysis of reported productivity losses, work changes, and leaving the labor force, *Arthritis Care & Research*, 59, 12: 1805–13.

Gulland, J. (2011), *Excessive sickness claims': controlling sickness and incapacity benefits in the early 20th century*, Paper given at the Social Policy Association annual conference, Lincoln, UK, 4–6 July.

Hansson, M., Bostrom, C. and Harms-Ringdahl, K. (2006), Sickness absence and sickness attendance – what people with neck or back pain think, *Social Science & Medicine*, 62: 2183–95.

Harrington, M. (2011), *An Independent Review of the Work Capability Assessment – Year Two*, London: The Stationery Office for the Department of Work and Pensions.

Hodgson, D. E. (2004), Project work: the legacy of bureaucratic control in the post-bureaucratic organization, *Organization*, 11, 1: 81–100.

Houston, D. and Lindsay, C. (2010), Fit for work? Health, employability and challenges for the UK welfare reform agenda, *Policy Studies*, 31, 2: 133–42.

Irvine, A. (2011), Fit for work? The influence of sick pay and job flexibility on sickness absence and implications for presenteeism, *Social Policy & Administration*, 45, 7: 752–69.

Johansson, G. and Lundberg, I. (2004), Adjustment latitude and attendance requirements as determinants of sickness absence or attendance. Empirical tests of the illness flexibility model, *Social Science & Medicine*, 58: 1857–68.

Jones, M. K. and Latreille, P. (2011), Disability and self-employment: evidence from the UK LFS, *Applied Economics*, 43, 27: 4161–78.

Kangas, O. (2010), Work accident and sickness benefits. In F. Castles (ed.), *Oxford Handbook of the Welfare State*, Oxford: Oxford University Press.

Karagiannaki, E. (2011), *The Magnitude and Correlates of Inter-vivos Transfers in the UK*, CASE paper 151, London: Centre for Analysis of Social Exclusion, London School of Economics.

Kemp, P. A., Sunden, A. and Tauritz, B. (2006), *Sick Societies? Trends in Disability Benefits in Post-industrial Welfare States*, Geneva: International Social Security Association.

Kennedy, F., Haslam, C., Munir, F. and Pryce, J. (2007), Returning to work following cancer: a qualitative exploratory study into the experience of returning to work following cancer, *European Journal of Cancer Care*, 16, 1: 17–25.

Liedberg, G. and Henriksson, C. (2002), Factors of importance for work disability in women with fibromyalgia: an interview study, *Arthritis Care & Research*, 47, 3: 266–74.

Longhi, S., Nicoletti, C. and Platt, L. (2009), *Decomposing wage gaps across the pay distribution: investigating inequalities of ethno-religious groups and disabled people*, ISER Working Paper No. 2009–3, Colchester: Institute for Social and Economic Research, University of Essex.

Maltby, T. (2011), Extending working lives? Employability, work ability and better quality working lives, *Social Policy and Society*, 10, 3: 299–308.

Manderbacka, K. (1998), How do respondents understand survey questions on ill-health? *European Journal of Public Health*, 8, 4: 319–24.

Maxwell, J. A. (2004), Using qualitative methods for causal explanation, *Field Methods*, 16, 3: 243–64.

McQuaid, R. W. and Lindsay, C. (2005), The concept of employability, *Urban Studies*, 42, 2: 197–219.

McVicar, D. (2006), Why do disability benefit rolls vary between regions? A review of the evidence from the USA and the UK, *Regional Studies*, 40, 5: 519–33.

McVicar, D. (2009), *Local Level Incapacity Benefits Rolls in Britain: Correlates and Convergence*, Belfast: Queen's University School of Management, Queen's University Belfast.

Organisation for Economic Co-operation and Development (OECD) (2003), *Transforming Disability into Ability: Policies to Promote Work and Income Security for Disabled People*, Paris: OECD.

Organisation for Economic Co-operation and Development (OECD) (2010), *Sickness, Disability and Work: Breaking the Barriers. A Synthesis of Findings across OECD Countries*, Paris, OECD.

Østby, K., Ørstavik, R., Knudsen, A., Reichborn-Kjennerud, T. and Mykletun, A. (2011), Health problems account for a small part of the association between socioeconomic status and disability pension award. Results from the Hordaland Health Study, *BMC Public Health*, 11: 12.

Palmer, K. and Cox, R. (2007), A general framework for assessing fitness for work. In K. Palmer, R. Cox and I. Brown (eds), *Fitness for Work: The Medical Aspects*, 4th edn, Oxford: Oxford University Press, pp. 1–20.

Ritchie, J. and Lewis, J. (2003), *Qualitative Research Practice: A Guide for Social Science Students and Researchers*, London: Sage.

Sainsbury, R. and Davidson, J. (2006), *Routes onto incapacity benefits: findings from qualitative research*, Department for Work and Pensions Research Report No 350, Norwich: HMSO.

Sainsbury, R., Irvine, A., Aston, J., Wilson, S., Williams, C. and Sinclair, A. (2008), *Mental health and employment*, Department for Work and Pensions Research Report No 513, Norwich: HMSO.

van den Berg, T. I. J., Elders, L. A. M., De Zwart, B. and Burdorf, A. (2009), The effects of work-related and individual factors on the Work Ability Index: a systematic review, *Occupational and Environmental Medicine*, 66: 211–20.

van Oorschot, W. (2006), Making the difference in social Europe: deservingness perceptions among citizens of European welfare states, *Journal of European Social Policy*, 16, 1: 23–42.

Wade, D. T. and Halligan, P. W. (2004), Do biomedical models of illness make for good healthcare systems? *British Medical Journal*, 329, 7479: 1398–401.

Wilton, R. D. (2008), Workers with disabilities and the challenges of emotional labour, *Disability & Society*, 23, 4: 361–73.

## Supporting Information

Additional supporting information may be found in the online version of this article at the publisher's website:

**Table S1** Anonymised list of participants

# 4

## 'Keeping meself to meself' – How Social Networks Can Influence Narratives of Stigma and Identity for Long-term Sickness Benefits Recipients

### Kayleigh Garthwaite

### Introduction

Since 2008, the UK has been experiencing a period of welfare reform and austerity which has caused increasing stigma, shame and uncertainty for many sickness benefits recipients. Briefly, Employment and Support Allowance (ESA) was initially introduced by Brown's Labour Government in 2008, and saw the attachment of work-related conditions to the receipt of sickness benefit (DWP 2008). The UK coalition Government adopted this approach, and under the ESA regime, new claimants must undergo the Work Capability Assessment (WCA), a health capacity test to determine their fitness for work. From April 2011, those claiming Incapacity Benefit (IB) started to undertake this assessment. Ongoing reform has, for example, led to research that has discussed the geographical distribution of welfare reform (Beatty and Fothergill 2014), the role of identity within the narratives of long-term sickness benefits recipients (Garthwaite 2015), fear over welfare reform (Garthwaite 2013), and conditionality (Patrick 2011; Weston 2012). Geographically, the work of Beatty and colleagues (also in this Special Issue) has repeatedly discussed how the highest claimant rates are nearly all found in Britain's older industrial areas – in the South Wales Valleys, in the North of England in places such as Merseyside, Lancashire, South Yorkshire, Teesside, Durham and Tyneside, and in the West of Scotland in and around Glasgow (Beatty and Fothergill 2014, 2013, 2005; Beatty et al. 2009). These are the parts of Britain where large-scale industrial job losses occurred in the 1980s and early 1990s where there has been a continuing imbalance between labour demand and labour supply.

*New Perspectives on Health, Disability, Welfare and the Labour Market*, First Edition.
Edited by Colin Lindsay, Bent Greve, Ignazio Cabras, Nick Ellison and Stephen Kellett.
© 2015 John Wiley & Sons, Ltd. Published 2015 by John Wiley & Sons, Ltd.

In the UK, the popular media have contributed significantly to a hardening of attitudes to welfare recipients in recent years, characterizing benefits recipients as 'scroungers', 'lazy', 'workshy' and 'fraudsters'. The accompanying policy shifts from an emphasis on universalism to one on conditionality and selectivity has reaffirmed this (Golding and Middleton 1982; Garthwaite 2011; Horton and Gregory 2009; Sefton 2009). Drawing on data collected during a qualitative study of long-term sickness benefits recipients in the North East of England, this article is particularly interested in how narratives of those receiving long-term sickness benefits are influenced and shaped by social networks in the form of friends, family, communities and employment, and how this relates to stigma and identity.

It can be argued that a stigma is essentially an attribute of the stigmatized person. A stigma is a mark of disgrace. The mark may be a physical one, or it may be something which attaches to the person, like a stain or taint. Goffman (1963) at first refers to stigma as 'a failing, a short-coming, a handicap' (Goffman 1963: 12); 'an attribute that is deeply discrediting' (Goffman 1963: 13); 'an attribute that makes him different from others ... and of a less desirable kind' (Goffman 1963: 12); and 'a shameful differentness' (Goffman 1963: 21). Goffman goes on to say that, 'a stigma ... is really a special kind of relationship between attribute and stereotype' (Goffman 1963: 14). These definitions present stigma as a personal flaw – and one which can be likened to the rhetoric surrounding benefits recipients as a result of media and government discourse. Using Goffman's (1967) notion of stigma management including 'saving face' and presenting an 'idealized self' (Goffman 1959), this article goes on to illustrate the different arenas within which stigma is co-constructed and how people receiving long-term sickness benefits are acutely aware of its potential emergence in everyday social interaction (Goffman 1963). In response, participants attempted to avoid stigma at all costs, by withdrawing from social interactions which might expose their claimant status or reveal to friends and family the extent of their health problems, leading to a compromising of their social networks.

## Methods

The research presented here is based on doctoral research which was attached to a wider project involving a longitudinal survey of the health of long-term IB recipients in County Durham (Warren *et al.* 2013). County Durham, the site for the research presented here, is a region replete with a coal mining legacy that relates to wider, long-term processes in the economy and regional labour market, some of the highest levels of sickness benefits receipt in the country have been recorded. Figures show that there were 8.4 per cent of the working age population receiving ESA and incapacity benefits in the County Durham region in 2013, significantly higher than the national average of 6.1 per cent. In the Horden North ward of the county, this figure rises to 16.8 per cent, with a further 14.3 per cent in Easington Colliery (NOMIS 2013). All participants were initially recruited via Jobcentre Plus (JCP) 'Choices' outreach events held between September 2009 and June 2010 in the North East of England, an area where levels of deprivation, ill health and health inequalities are well pronounced. The Choices events aimed to offer a range of new and existing provision available at JCP and offered to people taking part in Pathways to Work, including initiatives such as the Condition Management Programme (CMP), Return to Work Credit and enhanced In-Work Support. Initial contact with participants was forged following attendance at the Choices events in venues such as local colleges, community centres, and leisure centres. JCP stated there was no compulsion for people to attend, and as the events were not mandatory, non-attendance would not impact upon someone's benefits receipt.

Purposive sampling was used to recruit 25 chronically ill and disabled people (15 women and ten men) who were interviewed between March 2011 and August 2011, with the majority of interviews taking place in participants' own homes. Importantly, participants involved in the research were all long-term IB recipients and were predominantly yet to undergo the WCA so therefore had not been migrated onto ESA or Jobseeker's Allowance at the time of the fieldwork. This should be kept in mind when references are made to IB or Disability Living Allowance throughout this article. Interviews lasted between 45 and 120 minutes and were transcribed verbatim and fully anonymized before thematic analysis was undertaken. The age range of the sample varied from 32 to 63. Only two participants reported growing up with health problems which were musculoskeletal in nature. Diagnoses most frequently reported included arthritis, rheumatism, fibromyalgia, cardiovascular disease, multiple sclerosis and mental health problems including depression and bipolar disorder. A substantial range existed between the lengths of time people had spent on IB – some had been receiving it for three years, whilst others had been receiving the benefit for over 20 years.

A thematic framework for analysis was derived partly from the study objectives and partly by identifying themes from ongoing analysis of transcripts. NVivo 8 software was also employed to assist with coding and to ensure transcripts had been analyzed thoroughly. All participants' names have been anonymized and any identifying information has been omitted. Ethical considerations were respected throughout the research and ethical clearance was approved in advance by Durham University Department of Geography Ethics Committee.

## Findings

### The importance of social networks – family and family

The importance of friends and family was a common theme throughout the narratives. Whilst for some, the support of those in their social networks was crucial in terms of their daily coping, for others, friends and family were shut out by participants who preferred to keep their health and illness narratives to themselves, often due to the stigma of being a benefits recipient.

*Case study: the Wellington Men's Group*

This discussion can be strengthened by looking at a case study example of the Wellington Men's Health Group. Originally set up through CMP, every Monday afternoon men with health problems in the Wellington area meet up to chat, tend to their allotments, plan what training courses they would like to do, arrange day trips and discuss any problems they may be facing, whether that may be in terms of health, benefits or other concerns. At each group, approximately eight to ten men typically in their 40s and 50s attend each week. Of particular importance here is the geographical work of Gesler (1992, 1993) on the notion of 'therapeutic landscapes'. Based on an understanding of the ways in which environmental, societal and individual factors can work together to preserve health and well-being, Gesler suggests that certain environments, in this case allotments, promote mental and physical well-being. Gesler's concept suggests that specific landscapes not only provide an identity but can also act as the location of social networks, providing settings for therapeutic activities. Furthermore, Milligan and colleagues (2004: 1787) discuss the importance of allotments and comment that such communal activity can have a positive impact upon health and well-being, but that, 'the benefits arising from the social interaction inherent within such communal gardening activity also have a powerful potential to address the UK government's social exclusion agenda'. These explanations fit neatly into the narratives of the three members of the group who were interviewed – Shaun, Fred and Ray – with all of them speaking of the significance the group has had in their lives. Fred, 53, had been receiving IB for over eight years. He used to be in the Army and had '*worked all of his life*' until polyarthritis left him unable to continue being employed. Fred was referred to the group through CMP five years ago. For Fred, the group not only allowed him to enjoy social activities such as day trips, but was also a source of information and support, '*They may have experienced something I haven't like with the benefits office and they can advise me. I've actually managed to help two ex-soldiers as well just sitting in the cafe talking to them*'. Ray struggled with alcoholism and for him the group was a way of giving his day '*more purpose*' and providing a structure that prevented him from beginning drinking alcohol at 3 pm:

> '*Ganning [going] to the men's group and doing stuff like this, I think if it wasn't for stuff like this I'd be stuck in the house a lot more. It's given us a bit purpose to get out. Being at the men's group there's a bit purpose cos you're meeting other people as well cos basically at the minute when I come here I'll start me drinking at 5, half 5. If I'm in the house not doing nowt I might kick off about 3.*'

Yet for Shaun, whilst he attends the group regularly, as the chairman he feels pressure to be the person who helps everyone else with their problems; as a result he feels his own concerns are being neglected. Shaun, 42, broke his back in an accident in his job as a bricklayer and now suffers with mental health problems after 13 years receiving sickness benefits:

> *'I've got the support group and I tried to talk to them and they said they see me as the one who sorts problems out. It's me strength that's kept me going all these years and I just feel like I'm running out of strength. They elected us chairman and I didn't even want to be elected, so I feel I've got a responsibility now when really I can't face it.'*

### Fractured relationships

Many participants spoke about how their relationships with family and friends had altered following their transition onto sickness benefits, characterized by a change in identity. When asked about friends and family, Mick said:

> *'I do miss socialising a lot, I can't do what I used to do but life goes on, friends come to see me as well, we have a chinwag but that friendship is different. The identity of the friendship has changed 'cos I can't do the things I used to do with them, the daft things we used to do, play football and we still have the same laughs and things but at work that history of all the daft things that happened, that's sort of slowly evaporating, those stored memories. Even though I've got friends the visits aren't what they used to be.'*

Nostalgia for a past identity was a theme which united the narratives. Mick spoke about his feelings of a loss of self and identity in relation to his friends – he feels things have changed between them. An equally told story was one of friends no longer visiting following the onset of chronic health problems. Shaun said:

> *'I was losing all me friends cos they felt uncomfortable coming round, they felt bad talking about what they were doing 'cos I couldn't do anything anymore. I decided I didn't want anything more to do with me sister after what she'd said about me [she wanted Shaun to be detained in a psychiatric hospital] and it was just horrendous.'*

Similarly, Martin, age 54, had been receiving IB for five years as a result of physical health problems and alcohol misuse. Martin described how his friends no longer visited him anymore, *'All our friends the only time we saw them was in the club, but now nobody visits us. But I'm quite content because over the years you just get used to it'*. Sue, 50, had been receiving IB for 20 years after an accident at work where she fell down a flight of stairs which led to mobility issues and depression. She is also diagnosed with diabetes and has heart problems. Sue spoke about the embarrassment she felt at asking her family for help:

> '*I think sometimes rightly or wrongly if I'm saying to the family "Me hands are bad" I think they must think "Oh she's off again" and I don't know whether they do but I think they must think I always complain. I dunno I've never actually asked them but I'm sure they must get sick of us saying can you do this, can you do that. They should n't have to be doing it. Like asking Catherine [daughter] to put me socks on, fasten me bra or put me knickers on up to here so I can pull them up – it's embarrassing. I know she'll do it but she shouldn't have to and that hurts.*'

These extracts suggest that suffering chronic illness can serve to isolate and separate people from their social networks, which could have a damaging effect upon their health; similar sentiments can be found in the work of Gallant *et al.* (2007) on family and friends in relation to chronic illness management.

Others such as Sandra chose not to fully share their problems with family and friends. Concealing identities and controlling information meant not only deciding who can be given information about their illness, but also how much and what information they would be given, thereby employing a form of stigma management (Goffman 1963). Just as there was an avoidance of accepting the term 'disabled', the stigma of receiving sickness benefits could be so overwhelming that people refused to admit they were receiving it (Garthwaite 2013). In some cases, interviewees refused to reveal their 'claimant identity' to close family and friends, and would avoid social situations to avoid being asked the question. Sandra, 45, was involved in a car accident 30 years ago which left her with spinal problems, and has since developed gastric problems alongside secondary mental health concerns. Sandra had received sickness benefits for 12 years but had not revealed this to anyone other than her husband, the relevant authorities and myself. Sandra described how friends and family can fail to understand the complexities of sickness and disability – something made even more difficult given the fact that Sandra refused to disclose her long-term sickness benefits recipient status:

> '*I bumped into a friend who I hadn't seen for 30 years and she asked if I was working and when I said no, she was like "Oh I wish I could be a lady of leisure, I wish I had nothing to do all day" and I thought you haven't got a clue. It's like my sister she works full time and I said to her I would love to be earning £300 a week, getting a pay packet, earning money – I would love to be in her shoes. But like I say they don't understand why I'm not working, they know I have back problems but nothing more.*'

There were numerous occasions where participants described avoiding social situations which risked exposing their claimant identity and would not admit to needing help because it would mean a loss of pride or face (Goffman 1967). Here, Sandra is actively distancing herself from friends and family members as she feels ashamed and concerned about others' reaction to her illness and benefit status. Employing the theoretical framing of Goffman to offer an explanation for Sandra's behaviour, the notion of 'idealized self' (Goffman 1959: 45) occurs 'when the individual presents himself before others … to incorporate and exemplify the officially credited values of the society'. Indeed, according to Goffman (1963: 42), the pressure of idealized conduct is most clearly seen in marginalized people, such as long-term sickness benefits recipients, who are viewed as 'discredited'.

## Stigma, Networks and the Community: 'keeping meself to meself'

Studies have emphasized the continued existence of strong, local social ties within disadvantaged neighbourhoods in diverse locations including the UK, Ireland and Australia (Gosling 2008; Leonard 2004; Olagnero *et al.* 2005; Warr 2005). These interactions can provide practical help (Gosling 2008; Warr 2005) as well as a sense of attachment and belonging to place (Robertson *et al.* 2008). Interestingly, when asked about their local area, very few participants reflected upon the history or the importance a place can have upon health. Instead, the answer people gave when asked about the area was the same time and time again – '*I keep meself to meself*'. This could be linked to wider feelings of shame and guilt related to receiving sickness benefits – as the findings presented here and elsewhere (Garthwaite 2013) suggest, people can be reluctant to reveal a 'claimant' identity to friends and family, so 'keeping meself to meself' can be perceived as an extension of that when thinking about place and community. A clear distinction between identifying as 'deserving' benefits recipients and those in the area who they perceived as 'undeserving' was apparent in the narratives. Angie, 50, had been receiving sickness benefits for over seven years following a serious car accident which led to both physical and mental health problems. She initially spoke of her perception that many people were receiving benefits in her neighbourhood, yet when she reflected on her comments, she realized that may not be the case:

'*Oh gosh yeah, even if they're not supposed to be. The girl who was living next door she's gone now but she was working a couple of jobs and then she was claiming as well and she got caught but I mean … although Amanda next door has jobs, the house at the end Stephanie she goes cleaning, Sally works with handicapped kids, next door they both work, the next door I think they work so … maybes y'know there's not that many. When you sit and think about it, maybe there aren't many on benefits here so it might not be that bad. But like I say I tend to keep meself to meself.*'

The importance of community was alluded to by several participants in the study, such as Linda and Mick, as shown in these extracts below. Linda, 54, had physical health problems which she attributed to working in factories for many years, together with mental health problems that developed following her exit from the labour market. Linda said, '*I like getting outside, getting out in the back lane when someone's out. We've had some laughs up here it was all community, a hell of a community. Like I say we always have little bonfires, parties … its great up here when it's like that*'.

## Welfare and the neighbourhood

In their study of attitudes to welfare recipients and neighbourhoods, Bailey *et al.* (2013) comment how living in a poorer neighbourhood could be associated with exposure to slightly less supportive attitudes and hence a weaker, negative effect on residents' attitudes. For Shaun, the downside of community could be found in his neighbours' attitudes towards him and his condition:

'*The amount of times I've heard the neighbours saying "He's supposed to be bad but look he's going out for the night" and I felt like turning round and saying "Hang on a minute" and I hate it, to the point where now that I've moved again to a different area I deliberately keep meself to meself*.'

Again, the quotation from Shaun's interview highlights how stigma encourages him to withdraw from social networks in his neighbourhood resulting in him 'keeping meself to meself'. Efforts to limit social contact with other residents were also evident in research by Crisp (2013). A number of residents in his study of disadvantaged neighbourhoods articulated a desire to 'keep themselves to themselves'. Crisp (2013) explains that tendencies to regulate contact with neighbours was expressed in terms of choice which can be seen as fitting into the ideas of 'community unbound'. This term refers to broad changes in the social and economic structure have reduced reliance on neighbours and encouraged a 'privatization of community' (Blokland 2003) which includes a growing preference for more intimate networks of family and friends.

On occasions, but not often, participants did talk about how the decline of the local labour market in County Durham and the North East had an impact upon their narratives. For example, Linda, explained how she felt her job prospects were being restricted and why, '*I couldn't work in a shop, petrol stations aren't the same, I haven't done anything else. All I've ever done is work in a factory since leaving school. There is no factories they're all shut, every one I've worked in has closed down, every single one*'. Joan, 52, reflects upon how the area has changed since it ceased to be a working pit village, '*It's not as lively an area as it used to be and there's clubs closing down, there's not a lot of shops open now, the library's gone it's now a car park*'.

Indeed, Cattell's work (2001: 1504) highlights how dwindling facilities like social clubs and local shops mean that there are fewer casual meeting places on the estates she studied than there once were, but those remaining continue to have significance for fostering the weak ties necessary for a vibrant community life and which her interviewees suggested contributed to their own sense of well-being as can be seen in

Linda's comments about '*getting out in the back lane*'. Although some participants were reluctant to engage with social networks, generally narratives revealed recognition of the benefits of employment not just financially, but socially, morally and for their health and well-being.

## Missing 'the craic': The Social Side of Working

Work constitutes a key part of how we construct, define, transform and make sense of our own and others' identities (Bain 2005). The social aspect of work was described as being incredibly important for participants, and something that was hugely missed following their transition onto long-term sickness benefits. This transition from paid employment was also instrumental in shaping current identities (Garthwaite 2015). Jennifer, 56, and her husband were both receiving sickness benefits. Jennifer had arthritis alongside severe mental health problems and a host of other physical health concerns and had been receiving sickness benefits for 12 years. Jennifer said, '*I would love to work, it's like you if it happened to you you'd think "I'm stuck what am I gonna do?" I bet when you have holidays you get frustrated and want to be back at work. It's social, socialising and we haven't got that no more*'. Talking about the importance of work to her, Linda was enthusiastic about how 'the *craic*' or social side of working in a factory was appealing to her:

> '*It was very important, I loved it. The girls, the craic, we had a hell of a laugh. Music on all day, singing, dancing, carrying on … it was one big laugh from start to finish. There's nothing like working in a factory I loved it, it was a blast. As long as you got your work done it didn't matter what you were doing, as long as you kept that line going. I loved it.*'

Angie's interview revealed a similar sentiment. For her, work was important due to the social aspect that accompanied it:

> '*I loved to work. I worked in the doctors we were all friends I had meals out, things like that. You know what it's like, you work. We used to go to London together, things like that and [when you come out of work] you lose everything, you lose your friends, you lose your job which I loved me job, I love people working with people and I just loved it all, I really did.*'

Both Jennifer and Angie were keen to stress how as the researcher, I am employed and would, like them, miss the social aspect of work if it was absent. This again reinforces the stigma they felt at being 'discredited' (Goffman 1963) and having to claim for sickness benefits. Kirsty, 33, a prison officer for ten years until an accident at work left her with permanent spinal problems, spoke of her concerns over the absence of work within her identity:

> '*The first question people always ask you after your name is "What do you do?" and it kind of defines you. I usually just say to people "I don't, I retired*

*when I was 30" and they give you a double take and wonder what the heck
you're going on about but yeah it does define what you do. People look at you
and think "There's bugger all wrong with you". I've had that conversation
so many times with people and you're having to justify why you don't have
a job. I would rather be able to turn around and say anything really rather
than that.'*

The problem with unemployment is not the lack of resources as such,
but the deprivation of the legitimate means by which resources are
secured by employed people and the demoralizing effect this has on
people 'in terms of a series of lacunae associated with a state of non-
working' (Walters 2000: 85), as can clearly be seen in Trevor's narrative.
Trevor, 59, was involved in a motorbike accident which left him with
neck and arm problems. He had been receiving sickness benefits for
nine years and said:

*'It was pretty tough 'cos I'd been doing that job for 30 years and to lose all
me friends, me contacts basically coming back home… although I classed it
as home it wasn't really 'cos I had no friends here, friends I'd grew up with
and served my time with in the ship yards I hadn't seen them for 20 odd
years. So… it was tough, psychologically tough. Then obviously once I was
capable and got me confidence back and came off all the drugs I was on I
got me confidence back, then I had to set about thinking "What am I gonna
do employment wise?" 'cos I had to get a job, I've always worked.'*

For Trevor, unemployment meant a state of deficit in relation to a set
of 'enduring human needs' that are provided for by paid work (Jahoda
1982: 60). Unemployment takes away shared experience; a structured
experience of time; collective purpose; required regular activity; and,
lastly, status and identity. 'What do you do?' remains a question strangers
wonder about each other when they meet. It is also important to view
the appeal of work in terms of a desire to avoid the shame and stigma
experienced due to the lack of it in an individual's narrative.

### Discussion and Conclusions

This article explores the processes that long-term sickness benefits recipients engaged with in order to negotiate stigma and identity in their
social networks. In particular, it seeks to contribute to discussions centred on attitudes to welfare recipients, communities and employment.

First, narratives were filled with isolation and exclusion which was
exacerbated by the negative discourse which surrounds sickness benefits receipt in populist media representations. As a result of this pejo-
rative discourse, together with burgeoning welfare reform, long-term
sickness benefits recipients can experience stigma that results in them
'keeping meself to meself' and therefore withdrawing from social networks and ties. Yet this ignores the complexity of life as a sickness benefits recipient in often disadvantaged communities. Indeed Baumberg

74

*et al.* (2012) suggest there is a genuine link between negative media coverage and stigma – although we can only fully appreciate the media's impact when we consider its inter-relationship with people's everyday experiences. This article shows that whilst the presence of friends and family may have positive influences upon an individual's narrative, they can also bring negative influences for the individual to contend with. One way of explaining this finding is to try to understand and appreciate the complexity of living in deprived communities such as those in the study. Research by O'Leary and Salter (2014) found that multiple disadvantage is a story of interdependence between people, not just between problems. In particular, families can provide a vital extra layer of resilience, helping people in ways and at times that statutory services cannot. Policy often does too little to take account of this interdependence. Policies can serve to actively undermine the kind of self-help and mutual support that families engage in. Reforms such as the removal of the under-occupancy penalty (the 'bedroom tax') have left people with the choice of either finding more money for rent or moving away from the support networks that make life liveable for many. On the other hand, and as the findings here have shown, fractured relationships with family and friends can diminish people's capacity to flourish (O'Leary and Salter 2014; MacDonald *et al.* 2005; Spano 2002).

Second, neighbourhoods are vulnerable to being stigmatized with implications for residents' social networks, experiences of social connectedness and opportunities for developing or accessing social capital. Airey (2003) describes how residents in her study actively constructed social problems in Kirkhead as being perpetrated by specific groups of (other) people in specific (other) places within the neighbourhood. Airey (2003) has also argued that neighbourhood reputation can lead to psychosocial stress through the experience of shame, despite attempts to resist being 'tarred with the same brush'. These kinds of concerns also reflect the findings of a recent study by Chase and Walker (2013), who suggest that shame as a result of poverty can have a destructive impact on social solidarity, as people are keen to distance themselves from the 'Other' who is poor and 'not like them'. In an area such as County Durham where levels of sickness benefit receipt are much higher than the national and county averages, people living in the area can stigmatize other benefits recipients as the 'Other', as shown in the example given by Angie, who believed there were many more people receiving benefits in her community than was actually the case. Research in deprived communities in Teesside shows similar findings; in order to engage in identification (with 'the ordinary') and disidentification (from 'the undeserving') participants created phantom Others; an 'underclass' situated financially, culturally, socially and morally below them (Shildrick and MacDonald 2013: 299). Bush and colleagues extend Goffman's (1963) notion of stigma beyond the individual to space and place, and illustrate how an area can gain a 'spoiled identity', or be 'discredited' with reference to several sources of stigma, including, health stigma and social stigma (Bush *et al.* 2001: 53). Furthermore, they argue that people living within a 'stigmatised place' can be discredited with the 'same characteristics as those attributed to the place where they live' (Bush *et al.* 2001: 52).

Third, the narratives of long-term sickness benefits recipients presented in this study reveal biographies which recognize the social importance of work. Of particular note here is how people's experience of the stigma of claiming sickness benefits and their nostalgia around employment clashes with the government and media rhetoric that suggests that many people make a 'lifestyle choice' to be on benefits. Pahl *et al.*'s (2007) study of attitudes towards inequality found that groupings were identified on the basis of orientation to work. Interviewees made moral distinctions between people who were *willing* to work, people who were *unable* to work, and people who were *not prepared to work*. Those not prepared to work were labelled 'scroungers', 'parasites' and 'work-shy'. According to Smith (2005), the pervasiveness of such discourses forces individuals on the margins of the labour market to strive to assert a positive identity by distancing themselves from others deemed less worthy within the same neighbourhood. This process of 'Othering' can help define the self and affirm identify whilst reducing the stigma associated with occupying particular social and spatial locations (Crisp 2013). This raises the question as to whether, in fact, the problem is not so much unemployment at all. Rather, the current conception of what qualifies as legitimate 'work' activity in policy, political and popular discourse is the problem. As long as this privileging of paid work remains central to the idea of the responsible citizen (Dean 2003; Dwyer 2010), then those unable to participate in 'jobs' in the formal labour market will remain at risk of exclusion and vilification. Perhaps a shift in what is accepted as work participation for all working-age adults might open up opportunities to address stigma, such as caring, volunteering and parenting, which aside from paid employment can also provide sickness benefits recipients an identity (Garthwaite 2015). For participants in this study, work was seen as bringing with it a social identity that was a source of pride and achievement, revealing an antithesis to the scrounger myth much popularized in the media, and perhaps reflecting the power of government rhetoric on the importance of paid work. There is quite clearly a visible link between how people construct work as being important, and how the government frames this in a very similar way. Such a framing by participants could be interpreted as an argument for a continuation of welfare-to-work activation policies; however, this would ignore the complex reality of welfare reform which brings stigma, isolation and suffering for those who are experiencing it.

## Acknowledgements

Thank you to the participants in the study who gave up their time to take part in the research. Thanks also to the editorial board and to the two very helpful anonymous reviewers. The project was funded by County

Durham and Darlington Primary Care Trust. The views expressed are those of the authors and not of the funders.

## References

Airey, L. (2003), Nae as nice a scheme as it used to be: lay accounts of neighbourhood incivilities and well-being, *Health & Place*, 9: 129–37.

Bailey, N., Gannon, M., Kearns, A., Livingston, M. and Leyland, A. H. (2013), Living apart, losing sympathy? How neighbourhood context affects attitudes to redistribution and to welfare recipients, *Environment and Planning A*, 45.

Bain, A. (2005), Constructing an artistic identity, *Work, Employment and Society*, 19, 1: 25–46.

Baumberg, B., Bell, K. and Gaffney, D. (2012), *Benefits Stigma in Britain*, London: Turn2Us.

Beatty, C. and Fothergill, S. (2005), The diversion from 'unemployment to 'sickness' across British regions and districts, *Regional Studies*, 39: 837–54.

Beatty, C. and Fothergill, S. (2013), Disability benefits in the UK: an issue of health or jobs? In D. Houston and C. Lindsay (eds), *Disability Benefits, Welfare Reform and Employment Policy*, London: Palgrave Macmillan.

Beatty, C. and Fothergill, S. (2014), The local and regional impact of the UK's welfare reforms, *Cambridge Journal of Regions, Economy and Society*, 7, 1: 63–79.

Beatty, C., Fothergill, S., Houston, D., Powell, R. and Sissons, P. (2009), *Women on Incapacity Benefits*, Centre for Regional Economic and Social Research, Sheffield Hallam University and Department of Geography, University of Dundee.

Blokland, T. (2003), *Urban Bonds*, Cambridge: Polity Press.

Bush, J., Moffatt, S. and Dunn, C. (2001), 'Even the birds round here cough': stigma, air pollution and health in Teesside, *Health & Place*, 7, 1: 47–56.

Cattell, V. (2001), Poor people, poor places, and poor health: the mediating role of social networks and social capital, *Social Science & Medicine*, 52: 1501–16.

Chase, E. and Walker, R. (2013), The co-construction of shame in the context of poverty: beyond a threat to the social bond, *Sociology*, 47, 4: 739–54.

Crisp, R. (2013), 'Communities with oomph'? Exploring the potential for stronger social ties to revitalise disadvantaged neighbourhoods, *Environment and Planning C: Government and Policy*, 31, 2: 324–39.

Dean, H. (2003), Re-conceptualising welfare-to-work for people with multiple problems and needs, *Journal of Social Policy*, 32, 3: 441–59.

Department for Work and Pensions (DWP) (2008), *Raising Expectations and Increasing Support: Reforming Welfare for the Future*, London: The Stationery Office.

Dwyer, P. (2010), *Understanding Social Citizenship: Issues for Policy and Practice*, 2nd edn, Bristol: Policy Press.

Gallant, M. P., Spitze, G. D. and Prohaska, T. R. (2007), Help or hindrance? How family and friends influence chronic illness self-management among older adults, *Research on Aging*, 29: 375–409.

Garthwaite, K. (2011), 'The language of shirkers and scroungers?' Talking about illness, disability and coalition welfare reform, *Disability and Society*, 26, 3: 369–72.

Garthwaite, K. (2013), Fear of the brown envelope: exploring welfare reform with long-term sickness benefits recipients, *Social Policy & Administration*, 48, 7: 782–98.

Garthwaite, K. (2015), Becoming incapacitated? Long-term sickness benefit recipients and the construction of stigma and identity narratives, *Sociology of Health & Illness*, doi: 10.1111/1467-9566.12168.

Gesler, W. (1992), Therapeutic landscapes: medical issues in light of the new cultural geography, *Social Science & Medicine*, 34, 7: 735-46.

Gesler, W. (1993), Therapeutic landscapes: theory and a case study of Epidauros, Greece, *Environment and Planning D: Society and Space*, 11: 171-89.

Goffman, E. (1959), *The Presentation of Self in Everyday Life*, New York, NY: Doubleday.

Goffman, E. (1963), *Stigma: Notes on the Management of Spoiled Identity*, Harmondsworth: Penguin.

Goffman, E. (1967), *Interaction Ritual: Essays on Face-to-Face Behavior*, Garden City, NY: Doubleday.

Golding, P. and Middleton, S. (1982), *Images of Welfare*, Oxford: Martin Robinson.

Gosling, V. K. (2008), 'I've always managed, that's what we do': social capital and women's experiences of social exclusion, *Sociological Research Online*, 13, 1, http:// www.socresonline.org.uk/13/1/1.html (accessed 10 February 2014).

Horton, T. and Gregory, J. (2009), *The Solidarity Society: Why We Can Afford to End Poverty, and How to do it with Public Support*, London: Fabian Society.

Jahoda, M. (1982), *Employment and Unemployment: A Social-Psychological Analysis*, Cambridge: Cambridge University Press.

Leonard, M. (2004), Bonding and bridging social capital: reflections from Belfast, *Sociology*, 38: 927-44.

MacDonald, R., Shildrick, T., Webster, C. and Simpson, D. (2005), Growing up in poor neighbourhoods: the significance of class and place in the extended transitions of 'socially excluded' young adults, *Sociology*, 39, 5: 873-91.

Milligan, C., Gatrell, A. and Bingley, A. (2004), 'Cultivating health': therapeutic landscapes and older people in northern England, *Social Science & Medicine*, 58, 9: 1781-93.

NOMIS (2013), *DWP Benefit Claimants – Area Comparison*, August 2013, http://www.nomisweb.co.uk/reports/lmp/ward/1308630513/subreports/casdwp_compared/report.aspx (accessed 25 March 2014).

Olagnero, M., Meo, A. and Corcoran, M. (2005), Social support networks in impoverished European neighbourhoods, *European Societies*, 7: 53-79.

O'Leary D., and Salter, J. (2014), *Ties that Bind*, London: DEMOS.

Pahl, R., Rose, D. and Spencer, L. (2007), *Inequality and Quiescence: A Continuing Conundrum*, Colchester: Institute for Social & Economic Research, University of Essex, http://www.iser.essex.ac.uk/publications/working-papers/iser/2007-22.pdf (accessed 25 March 2014).

Patrick, R. (2011), Disabling or enabling: the extension of work related conditionality to disabled people, *Social Policy and Society*, 10, 3: 309-20.

Robertson, D., Smyth, J. and McIntosh, I. (2008), *Neighbourhood Identity, People, Time and Place*, York: Joseph Rowntree Foundation.

Sefton, T. (2009), Moving the right direction? Public attitudes to poverty, inequality and redistribution. In J. Hills, T. Sefton and K. Stewart (eds), *Towards a More Equal Society? Poverty, Inequality and Policy Since 1997*, Bristol: Policy Press, pp. 223-44.

Shildrick, T. and MacDonald, R. (2013), Poverty talk: how people experiencing poverty deny their poverty and why they blame 'the poor', *The Sociological Review*, 61, 2: 285-303.

Smith, D. (2005), *On the Margins of Inclusion: Changing Labour Markets and Social Exclusion in London*, Bristol: Policy Press.

Spano, A. (2002), Premodernity and postmodernity in Southern Italy, *Biography and Social Exclusion in Europe*, 61–76.

Walters, W. (2000), *Unemployment and Government: Genealogies of the Social*, Cambridge: Cambridge University Press.

Warr, D. J. (2005), Social networks in a 'discredited neighbourhood, *Journal of Sociology*, 41: 285–308.

Warren, J., Bambra, C., Kasim, A., Garthwaite, K., Mason, J. and Booth, M. (2013), Prospective evaluation of the effectiveness and cost utility of a pilot 'health first' case management service for long term Incapacity Benefit recipients, *Journal of Public Health*, 36, 1: 117–25.

Weston, K. (2012), Debating conditionality for disability benefits recipients and welfare reform: research evidence from Pathways to Work, *Local Economy*, 27, 5–6: 514–28.

# 5

## *Measuring the Impacts of Health Conditions on Work Incapacity – Evidence from the British Household Panel Survey*[*]

### William Whittaker[**] and Matt Sutton

### Introduction

The number of people claiming incapacity and disability benefits[1] (DB) in Great Britain has increased by over 300 per cent in 30 years (McVicar and Anyadike-Danes 2008). In 2013, DB claimants represented 6.1 per cent of the working-age population (NOMISWEB 2014a). During a period of stable rates of claiming DBs throughout the late 1990s and early 2000s, the proportion of claims for mental and behavioural disorders rose from 27 per cent in 1997 to 41 per cent in 2007 (NOMISWEB 2014b). These rises in claiming DBs are at odds with general improvements in health (Macnicol 2013). Claiming DBs can have a negative effect on an individual's health, particularly where an individual claims DBs over a long period (Bambra 2011); and may hinder future job prospects (Green and Shuttleworth 2013). In addition to offering fiscal benefits to the government and income benefits to the individual, moving into work from claiming benefits can have a positive impact on physical health and well-being (Waddell and Burton 2006; Black 2008).

Policymakers have responded to high rates of DB claimants by focusing on the behavioural aspects of individuals. Such policies have included the tightening and more acute monitoring of eligibility. For example, the introduction of the Welfare Reform Act 2007 in 2008 saw the Employment and Support Allowance (ESA) replace Incapacity Benefit (IB) for new claimants of DBs. The defining difference between the two benefits lies in the assessment of an individual's ability to be active in the labour market. Under IB, individuals had a Personal Capability Assessment (PCA), this was replaced with a Work Capability Assessment (WCA) under ESA. The WCA assesses an individual's ability to work in

*New Perspectives on Health, Disability, Welfare and the Labour Market*, First Edition.
Edited by Colin Lindsay, Bent Greve, Ignazio Cabras, Nick Ellison and Stephen Kellett.
© 2015 John Wiley & Sons, Ltd. Published 2015 by John Wiley & Sons, Ltd.

his or her current health state, whilst the PCA assessed an individual's ability to perform everyday tasks. Associated with the WCA, a Capability Report could also be issued which reports the help and support an individual may need to return to work.

The WCA marked a shift to more stringent medical assessments for DB eligibility. Additional policies have also focused on the individual as the 'problem', Pathways to Work (PtW), a scheme rolled out in the UK in 2008, aimed at enabling transitions to employment for those claiming DBs and centred around addressing deficiencies of the individual as a potential employee rather than the ability of employers to accommodate an individual's health condition. Such schemes remain today under the Work Programme whereby contractors are incentivized to move DB claimants into employment via a payment-by-results mechanism. The Work Programme has so far shown limited success in outcomes (Rees *et al.* 2014). Evidence has shown that the PtW scheme offered the potential to improve health and employment outcomes where employment-focused bodies worked in conjunction with healthcare providers (Kellett *et al.* 2011; Purdie and Kellett 2015). However, healthcare providers have had limited input into the Work Programme (Ceolta-Smith *et al.* 2015).

Over the period of these policy changes the number of individuals claiming DBs has reduced by approximately 200,000 (from 2.6 million in 2007 [6.8 per cent of the working age population] to 2.4 million in 2013 [6.1 per cent of the working age population]) (NOMISWEB 2014a).

For policies to be effective in reducing DB rates it is vital to understand the determinants of claiming DBs. As it is the main criteria for eligibility for DBs, understanding the influence of health is the most obvious starting point. This will enable a better design of health-specific interventions that may reduce the claiming of DBs.

There is a wide literature on the determinants of claiming DBs. Most studies have been cross-sectional (Disney and Webb 1991; Nolan and Fitzroy 2003; McVicar 2006; Barnes and Sissons 2013; Beatty *et al.* 2000, 2009, 2010, 2013) and/or have used aggregate data (Molho 1989, 1991; Holmes and Lynch 1990; Lynch 1991). Both approaches are limited in their ability to reveal the causal pathway between health and the claiming of DBs.

Consideration of only cross-sectional data means that dynamic modelling of claiming DBs is not possible. Dynamic modelling is important should claiming DBs be persistent. We believe claiming DBs is likely to be persistent for two reasons. First, claiming may be for a long-term health condition that may make claiming DBs a long-term state. Second, whilst individuals initially qualify for DBs on the basis of an existing health problem, claiming DBs may result in a worsening of that health problem, and/or generation of additional problems (particularly mental health). Both sources of persistence mean that cross-sectional associations between health and claiming DBs may overstate the effect that an individual's recovery back to full health (or enabling the individual to become active in the labour market with their condition) may have on transitions out of claiming DBs.

Aggregate (typically regional level) models of claiming DBs are also problematic since the inability to control for individual specific factors may lead to overestimation of the effects of health on claiming DBs.

Another limitation of past studies has been the lack of detailed data on health conditions. Molho (1989, 1991) proxied health via claiming of sickness benefits in a study using Department for Health and Social Services data. Disney and Webb (1991) used smoking status as the health measure in a study using the Family Expenditure Survey. Faggio and Nickell (2005) and McVicar and Anyadike-Danes (2008) both used self-reported disability. Two studies have examined the main health reason for claiming DBs from administrative data. Holmes and Lynch (1990) and Lynch (1991) found that the main health reason for claiming DBs had a significant effect on off-flows in the 1980s. Survey data from a sample of DB claimants have also found health to be the main reason for transitions into DB (Beatty *et al.* 2010, 2013). Where the main reason for claiming DBs have been modelled, these studies have not explicitly controlled for any potential confounding of the effects of other health problems. Two-thirds of DB claimants were found to have multiple health problems (Barnes and Sissons 2013). This type of confounding could have important implications for policy, as it may lead to over- or underestimation of the likelihood that individuals with resolved health problems will return to be active in the labour force.

To identify the causal pathway between health and claiming DBs, it is important to account for additional factors that may be correlated with health. Beatty *et al.* (2000) highlight the concepts of 'hidden unemployment' and 'hidden sickness' – processes by which labour market conditions and the relative values of unemployment and DB payments create incentives for the unemployed with (eligible) health conditions to transfer to DBs where unemployment is high and vice versa when unemployment is low. From the government's perspective this helps to reduce the numbers who are officially recorded as unemployed. From the individual perspective the claimant receives a higher benefit payment. A large volume of evidence exists showing rates of claiming DBs are higher in those areas most affected by de-industrialization (Beatty *et al.* 2000, 2009, 2010, 2013; Lindsay and Houston 2011; Webster *et al.* 2013).

This article aims to more accurately identify the causal pathway between health and claiming DBs by addressing several of the modelling problems present in the existing literature. We use nationally representative, individual-level, longitudinal survey data from the British Household Panel Survey (BHPS) to model influences on the probability of claiming DBs. The longitudinal nature of the data enables us to test whether the probability of claiming DBs is dynamic. Dynamic modelling of claiming DBs reduces the endogeneity problems generated by reverse causality between health and claiming DBs. We also include multiple health conditions in the model to allow us to control for confounding of the estimated effects of particular health conditions. To test for effects of the local labour market conditions, we include local unemployment and wage rates. Our analysis also controls for unobserved heterogeneity between individuals in the probability of claiming DBs and controls for several observed individual characteristics that may confound the (unconditional) effects of health.

## Data

We use data from the BHPS for the period 1991–2008 (University of Essex 2010a). The BHPS was an annual survey of each adult (16+) member of a nationally representative sample of more than 5,000 households. The same individuals are re-interviewed in successive waves and, if they split-off from original households, all adult members of their new households are also interviewed. Children are interviewed once they reach the age of 16. Thus the sample remains broadly representative of the population of Britain as it changes through time (Taylor *et al.* 2010).

The BHPS was superseded by Understanding Society in 2009. Although the Understanding Society sample incorporates BHPS respondents, we cannot include this data since harmonization of the two questionnaires resulted in the loss of several of the key variables in our analysis.

DB claimants are measured using the variable *f125*, which asks respondents: 'Have you yourself (or jointly with others) since 1st September last year received Incapacity Benefit?'. There are several important points to note here. First, this measure is retrospective. Second, the timing of interviews in the BHPS varies and as such the period covered by the question varies across observations. Third, this measure does not provide information on the number or duration of claim spells. Fourth, although claiming may be jointly with a partner, the benefits section of the BHPS questionnaire forms part of the individual income section of the BHPS questionnaire so it is unlikely respondents report claiming DBs when only their partner does. IB replaced Invalidity Benefit and Sickness Benefit in 1995. We code those claiming Invalidity Benefit and/or Sickness Benefit (*f117* and *f134* in the BHPS) in 1991–94 as DB claimants.

We restrict our sample to those of working age. We include women aged 16–59 years, and men aged 16–64 years at the time of the interview.

Given a high proportion of DB claims are coded as being due to mental and behavioural disorders, we initially only include depression as the measure of health. Depression is measured using the variable *hlprbi*, which asks respondents: 'Do you have any of the health problems or disabilities listed on this card. ... One of the listed conditions is 'Anxiety, depression or bad nerves'.

An alternative measure of mental health included in the BHPS is the 12-question version of the General Health Questionnaire (GHQ-12) which has been shown to be a valid measure of mental illness (Goldberg *et al.* 1997). We replicate our analysis with the 'caseness' definition of this variable, with individuals reporting a score of 4 or more (from a scale of 0 to 12) defined as having mental ill-health. Using data from a World Health Organization study across 15 countries, Goldberg *et al.* (1997) assess the validity of GHQ-12 as an indicator of current depression, dysthymia, agoraphobia, panic disorder, generalized anxiety disorder, somatization disorder, neurasthenia and hypchondriasis. These were measured using the ICD-10 (WHO 1990), and DSM-IV (APA 1994), with and without anxiety, and with and without alcohol dependence. The mean area under the Receiver Operating Characteristic curves was 0.88, overall sensitivity was 83.4 per cent and specificity 76.3 per cent. The average threshold across all centres was 2/3. Use of the binary measure of caseness enables a direct comparison of whether our results are robust to the measure of mental health used.

To assess the impact of confounding by other health conditions, we then include ten additional self-reported health measures. These follow the same format as depression but relate to problems with: arms and legs; sight; hearing; skin; chest; heart and blood; stomach; diabetes; epilepsy; and migraines.

We measure socio-economic group differences using the Registrar General's Social Class. The manual social class comprises skilled, partly-skilled and unskilled manual workers and the armed forces. Where the individual is unemployed, his or her last occupation is recorded. If there is no information on the individual's employment (e.g. if the individual has never worked) then we use the head of the household's occupation status, the father's occupation status, or the mother's occupation status in respective order.

The strength of the local labour market may also have an impact on the probability of claiming DBs. Job destruction, where people find themselves out of work, can be measured by the unemployment rate for the area. A high unemployment rate may encourage higher DB claiming rates, and those with health problems may be more likely to transit onto DBs once becoming unemployed. This can be described in two ways (Beatty *et al.* 2000):

1. the redundancy effect, whereby people of poorer health are more likely to be made redundant; and
2. the benefit shift, whereby people of poorer health are seen as relatively unattractive to employers compared to the healthy unemployed and are persistently sent to the back of the job queue as new waves of people enter unemployment.

In both cases, those in poorer health that qualify for DBs may switch to DBs as it pays higher than unemployment benefit. To capture variations in the strength of the local labour market, we utilize Local Authority District (LAD) level data on unemployment rates and average wage rates. This information was obtained from the claimant count (ONS 2014b), and the Annual Survey of Hours and Earnings (ONS 2014a), via NOMISWEB (NOMISWEB 2014c). LAD identifiers for the BHPS were provided by Data-Archive (University of Essex 2010b). Average wage rates are included to proxy the replacement rate of DB rates to local wages. As DB rates are national rates, the average regional wage captures regional differences in the relative financial value of DB payments.

## Methods

There are two important methodological concerns with modelling claiming DBs and depression. First, there are likely to be individual characteristics that are not measured in the BHPS which influence whether someone claims DBs, including attitudes to health and/or work. These unobserved characteristics are likely to be correlated with the variables in our model. For example, all else equal, earlier generations are more reluctant to claim financial benefits from the state (Costigan *et al.* 1999; Kotecha *et al.* 1999), which would exert negative bias on the estimated age gradient. Second, claiming DBs is likely to be persistent as claims for ill health may persist for a number of years for those with long-term health conditions. It is important to remove any correlation between the dependent variable and the error term for our estimates to be unbiased.

We follow Wooldridge (2005) in estimating a dynamic probit model with unobserved effects:

$$y_{it+1} = \beta_0 + \beta_1 z_{it} + \beta_3 y_{it} + c_i + u_{it} \tag{1}$$

The measure for claiming DBs in the BHPS is a binary indicator for whether an individual claimed DBs within the past year. $y_{it+1}$ identifies whether the individual claims DBs in the next year (BHPS variable $f125$ at $t + 1$). This ensures that current characteristics are not assigned to past claiming DBs. $y_{it}$ is a binary indicator for whether the individual claimed DBs in the past year. Modelling claiming DBs next year as the dependent variable means the maximum age modelled in the data is 59 for females and 64 for males. $c_i$ is an individual specific time-invariant error term that we allow to be correlated with $z_{it}$, a vector of covariates. $z_{it}$ contains dummy variables for other health problems and a range of variables found to be significant predictors for claiming DBs in the literature: age, region of residence, education, ethnic group, marital status, number of children, socio-economic group, area wage and unemployment rates, and survey year.

$z_{it}$ also contains an indicator for the recall period for the individual. This is the difference in days between the start of the recall period (1 September of the previous year) and the interview date. This controls for the possibility that individuals with longer recall periods have a longer period during which to have been at risk of claiming DBs.

Following Wooldridge (2005), we relax the (strong) assumption of zero heterogeneity by modelling $c_i$ as a function of: an initial condition, $y_{io}$ which is a binary variable indicating whether individual $i$ reported

86

having claimed DBs in their first observation, time-averages of the covariates, $\bar{z}_i$; and individual random-effects, $a_i$:

$$c_i|y_{io}, \bar{z}_i \sim Normal\left(\alpha_o + \alpha_1 y_{io} + \bar{z}_i\alpha_2, \sigma_a^2\right) \tag{2}$$

with:

$$c_i = \alpha_o + \alpha_1 y_{io} + \bar{z}_i\alpha_2 + a_i \text{ where } a_i|\left(y_{io}, \bar{z}_i\right) \sim Normal\left(0, \sigma_a^2\right)$$

The first additional term, $y_{io}$, is included in recognition that our sample is left-truncated, meaning we have no information on an individual's claiming DBs history before they enter the survey. $y_{io}$ is included since the first observation contains information on the unobserved tendency for an individual to claim DBs. The second set of additional terms is $\bar{z}_i$ which, like fixed-effects models, control for unobserved heterogeneity between individuals that is correlated with the time-averages of the covariates in the model. This removes correlation between the heterogeneity term and $z_{it}$ and therefore gives unbiased estimates on the coefficients of $z_{it}$. The third additional term, $a_i$, assumes a time-invariant individual-specific random-effects specification.

Substituting (2) into (1) gives:

$$y_{it+1} = \beta_o + \beta_1 z_{it} + \beta_2 y_{io} + \beta_3 y_t + \beta_4 \bar{z}_i + a_i + u_{it} \tag{3}$$

The difference between this dynamic random-effects model and a standard random-effects probit model is the inclusion of additional terms $y_{it}$, $y_{io}$ and $z_i$. It assumes that:

1. having conditioned on the covariates and unobserved heterogeneity, $z_{it}$ and $c_i$; the dynamics are correctly specified as first order;
2. $c_i$ is additive in the standard normal cumulative distribution function; and
3. the $z_{it}$ are strictly exogenous.

### Empirical strategy

We estimate several specifications of equation (3) to show the effects of controlling for each potential source of bias. First, we estimate a model for claiming DBs with depression as the only independent variable using a pooled probit regression to estimate the unconditional association between depression and claiming of DBs. Depression is chosen as our exemplar given the large proportion of DB claimants reporting mental health as the reason for claiming DBs. Second, we include individual characteristics to assess the impact of observed characteristics on the depression estimate. Depression is likely to be correlated with several of the additional characteristics (perhaps picking up age effects for example should older ages be both more likely to claim DBs and

87

more likely to report depression) and as such, expect the estimate for depression to vary once additional controls are added. Third, we control for unobserved characteristics that are assumed to be uncorrelated with the observed characteristics (perhaps identifying personality traits), this is performed using random-effects. Fourth, we control for dynamic DB claiming which may affect our estimated depression effect should those claiming DBs in the past be more likely to be depressed. Lastly, we model the final specification (equation (3)) where time averages of the covariates are included to control for correlation between the unobserved effect and the covariates (perhaps due to positive minded individuals being less likely to claim DB and less likely to report being depressed).

We estimate further specifications of equation (3) to check for the robustness of our results. First, the inclusion of the local wage and unemployment rates reduce the sample due to data availability, so we re-estimate equation (3) on this reduced sample without the local wage and unemployment rates to check whether any change in the results is due to the different sample. Second, as an alternative measure of mental health we model equation (3) replacing depression with GHQ caseness. Third, we estimate equation (3) using only those observed in each wave of the BHPS (the balanced sample) to gauge whether attrition may bias our estimates.

Following the literature (Molho 1989, 1991; Holmes and Lynch 1990; Lynch 1991; McVicar and Anyadike-Danes 2008), we estimate separate models for males and females. The models are estimated using *xtprobit, re* in STATA v13.0.

In order to interpret the magnitude of the estimates in equation (3), average marginal effects need to be estimated. These give the change in probability associated with a change in the covariate averaged across each observation. The average marginal effects are calculated using STATA's *margins* command, with the random effect assigned the mean value of zero and standard errors calculated using the delta method.

## Results

The initial sample of working age adults is 187,301 person-year observations (27,395 individuals). Use of one period lead values of DB claimant status reduces the sample to 162,569 observations (22,316 individuals). Item non-response on the remaining covariates results in a final sample of 150,661 person-year observations, comprising 72,337 observations for males and 78,324 observations for females (10,368 male individuals and 10,843 female individuals). Our panel is unbalanced and individuals can enter or leave the sample at any wave.

Table 1 compares the proportion of the working age population claiming IB and the proportion of claimants claiming for mental health problems from national administrative data, with the proportions of DB claimants in the BHPS reporting problems with depression and GHQ caseness. DBs can be claimed either as financial payment and/or

Table 1

Proportions of Disability Benefit claimants with mental health problems – comparison of administrative data with British Household Panel Survey Disability Benefit claiming and self-reported depression

| | Administrative data | | | | BHPS rates | | |
|---|---|---|---|---|---|---|---|
| Year | % working age claiming IB/SDA | % IB/SDA claims for mental and behavioural disorders | % working age claiming IB/SDA payments | % IB/SDA claims for mental and behavioural disorders | % working age claiming DBs | % DB claimants reporting depression as a health problem | % DB claimants with GHQ caseness |
| 1999 | 7.3 | 31.0 | 5.2 | 26.7 | 5.1 | 32.2 | 48.1 |
| 2000 | 7.4 | 32.3 | 5.2 | 27.8 | 5.2 | 36.9 | 45.1 |
| 2001 | 7.5 | 33.8 | 5.2 | 29.1 | 5.2 | 39.9 | 49.7 |
| 2002 | 7.4 | 35.5 | 5.0 | 30.4 | 4.9 | 39.2 | 48.6 |
| 2003 | 7.4 | 36.9 | 4.9 | 31.7 | 4.8 | 38.2 | 46.2 |
| 2004 | 7.4 | 38.3 | 4.8 | 32.8 | 5.1 | 40.8 | 45.0 |
| 2005 | 7.1 | 39.5 | 4.6 | 33.8 | 4.6 | 42.0 | 47.5 |
| 2006 | 7.0 | 40.5 | 4.4 | 34.7 | 4.5 | 42.2 | 47.2 |
| 2007 | 6.8 | 41.5 | 4.2 | 35.6 | 4.5 | 47.4 | 50.1 |

*Source*: administrative data from the DWP via NOMISWEB (NOMISWEB 2014b) (5% sample of National Insurance records for Great Britain).
*Note*: figures are for working-age adults only; working age is $> = 16$ and $< = 64$; SDA = Severe Disablement Allowance.

Table 2

Contingency table for depression and Incapacity Benefit claimant status

| | Respondent does not claim DBs in the next period | Respondent claims DBs in the next period | Total |
|---|---|---|---|
| **Males** | | | |
| Respondent is not depressed in the current wave | 66,016 (95.82) [96.51] | 2,879 (4.18) [73.13] | 68,895 (100.00) [95.24] |
| Respondent is depressed in the current wave | 2,384 (69.26) [3.49] | 1,058 (30.74) [26.87] | 3,442 (100.00) [4.76] |
| Total | 68,400 (94.56) [100.00] | 3,937 (5.44) [100.00] | 72,337 (100.00) [100.00] |
| **Females** | | | |
| Respondent is not depressed in the current wave | 68,952 (97.44) [91.71] | 1,812 (2.56) [57.76] | 70,764 (100.00) [90.35] |
| Respondent is depressed in the current wave | 6,235 (82.47) [8.29] | 1,325 (17.53) [42.24] | 7,560 (100.00) [9.65] |
| Total | 75,187 (95.99) [100.00] | 3,137 (4.01) [100.00] | 78,324 (100.00) [100.00] |

*Note:* cells contain: frequency (row percentage) and [column percentage].

National Insurance credits. As the question for claiming DBs forms part of the income section of the BHPS, respondents are likely to be reporting financial payments. The proportion of DB claimants in the BHPS is close to the population rate receiving payment and follows a similar trend. The rates claiming DBs and reporting problems with depression in the BHPS are higher than the national figures and the proportion with GHQ caseness even greater. Although the trend in depression follows a similar trend to the administrative data, GHQ caseness is more erratic.

Table 2 provides summary statistics on rates of depression and claiming DBs in the next period. For females there is a higher prevalence of depression than claiming DBs. Higher rates of illness than claiming DBs is not unusual. Sly *et al.* (1999) report 3.2 million people were active in the labour market though eligible for DBs in 1998/99 (for a discussion on these 'hidden sick', see Beatty *et al.* 2000).

Approximately 27 per cent of men and 42 per cent of women who claim DBs in the next period are depressed. While depression is more prevalent for women, depression appears to have a much stronger effect on claiming DBs in the next period for males. In the next period, 31 per cent of depressed males claim DBs compared with 4 per cent of non-depressed males. The equivalent figures are 18 per cent and 3 per cent for females. These effects are subject to significant bias as indications of the causal relationship between depression and claiming DBs.

Our first step to removing potential bias in the effects of depression on claiming DBs is to estimate a pooled OLS regression with the full set of covariates included. Table 3 provides average values of the covariates. There is a clear distinction between the prevalence of health conditions amongst males and females. Arms or legs, skin, chest/breathing, epilepsy, migraines and stomach/liver/kidney problems are all of a higher prevalence in females than males. Males have higher rates of problems related to sight, hearing, heart/blood and diabetes.

The results from multivariate analyses are provided in tables 4 and 5 for males and females, respectively. The estimates are reported as average marginal effects. In the first column of results, being depressed increases the probability of claiming DBs in the next wave by 12.5 percentage points for males and 8.0 percentage points for females. The results in the pooled with covariates model suggest a lower but still strongly significant positive effect of reporting depression on the probability of claiming DBs in the next wave. Univariate associations between depression and claiming DBs are in part identifying other factors that are both positively correlated with being depressed and with claiming DBs.

Our next stage in identifying causality between health and claiming DBs is to remove any bias generated by unobserved heterogeneity (unmeasured characteristics of individuals that may explain variations in claiming DBs). The third sets of results are from the static random-effects specification. The estimated effect of depression is significantly reduced to 1.4 percentage points for males and 0.7 percentage points for females.

To better identify the causal pathway between depression and claiming DBs, the model is then made dynamic, this reduces any concerns that the estimated effect of depression reflects current claiming DBs status. The fourth set of results is from the dynamic random-effects specification, which includes the lagged value of DB claimant status and the initial observed DB status. Both terms are highly significant for both genders and imply persistence in claiming DBs.

Our final model relaxes the assumption in random-effects models of zero correlation between the unmeasured characteristics and the covariates in the model. The fifth set of results are from the full dynamic model including the averages of the time-varying variables (equation (3)). These average values are jointly significant for both males and females. The estimated coefficients on the time-averages of the depression variable are positive and significant for both genders. Since this controls for any correlation of the unobserved heterogeneity with the proportion of waves in which the respondent reports depression, we are unable to disentangle the effect of long(er)-term depression from unobserved

Table 3

Descriptive statistics for covariates

| | Males | | Females | |
|---|---|---|---|---|
| | (N) | (%) | (N) | (%) |
| Total | 72,337 | 100.00 | 78,324 | 100.00 |
| Ethnic minority | | | | |
| No (base) | 67,124 | 92.79 | 72,736 | 92.87 |
| Yes | 5,212 | 7.21 | 5,588 | 7.13 |
| Age | | | | |
| 16–20 (base) | 7,316 | 10.11 | 7,932 | 10.13 |
| 21–25 | 6,869 | 9.50 | 7,726 | 9.86 |
| 26–30 | 7,785 | 10.76 | 9,260 | 11.82 |
| 31–35 | 8,690 | 12.01 | 10,448 | 13.34 |
| 36–40 | 8,823 | 12.20 | 10,485 | 13.39 |
| 41–45 | 8,304 | 11.48 | 9,692 | 12.37 |
| 46–50 | 7,527 | 10.41 | 8,923 | 11.39 |
| 51–55 | 6,940 | 9.59 | 8,065 | 10.30 |
| 56–59 | 4,880 | 6.75 | 5,793 | 7.40 |
| 62–64 | 5,203 | 7.19 | – | – |
| Children | | | | |
| None (base) | 44,599 | 61.65 | 42,233 | 53.92 |
| 1 | 13,544 | 18.72 | 17,827 | 22.76 |
| 2 | 10,296 | 14.23 | 13,104 | 16.73 |
| 3+ | 3,898 | 5.39 | 5,160 | 6.59 |
| Health problem | | | | |
| Arms or legs | 14,245 | 19.69 | 15,937 | 20.35 |
| Sight | 2,245 | 3.10 | 2,390 | 3.05 |
| Hearing | 4,312 | 5.96 | 2,676 | 3.42 |
| Skin | 6,809 | 9.41 | 11,595 | 14.80 |
| Chest, breathing | 7,726 | 10.68 | 9,237 | 11.79 |
| Heart and blood | 6,953 | 9.61 | 6,387 | 8.15 |
| Stomach, liver, kidney | 4,078 | 5.64 | 5,195 | 6.63 |
| Diabetes | 1,726 | 2.39 | 1,180 | 1.51 |
| Epilepsy | 561 | 0.78 | 662 | 0.85 |
| Migraine | 3,189 | 4.41 | 10,269 | 13.11 |
| Other | 1,914 | 2.65 | 4,015 | 5.13 |
| Marital status | | | | |
| Married (base) | 40,411 | 55.86 | 43,064 | 54.98 |
| Couple | 9,167 | 12.67 | 10,099 | 12.89 |
| Widowed | 489 | 0.68 | 1,257 | 1.60 |
| Divorced | 2,764 | 3.82 | 5,422 | 6.92 |
| Single | 19,506 | 26.97 | 18,482 | 23.60 |
| Region | | | | |
| London (base) | 4,937 | 6.82 | 5,360 | 6.84 |
| South East | 10,465 | 14.47 | 11,365 | 14.51 |
| South West | 5,042 | 6.97 | 5,238 | 6.69 |
| East Anglia | 2,264 | 3.13 | 2,348 | 3.00 |

Table 3

(*Continued*)

| | Males | | Females | |
|---|---|---|---|---|
| | (N) | (%) | (N) | (%) |
| Region (*cont.*) | | | | |
| East Midlands | 5,006 | 6.92 | 4,935 | 6.30 |
| West Midlands | 4,704 | 6.50 | 5,010 | 6.40 |
| North West | 5,761 | 7.96 | 6,100 | 7.79 |
| Yorks. & Humber. | 5,158 | 7.13 | 5,532 | 7.06 |
| North East | 3,486 | 4.82 | 3,502 | 4.47 |
| Wales | 9,013 | 12.46 | 9,697 | 12.38 |
| Scotland | 10,805 | 14.94 | 12,083 | 15.43 |
| Northern Ireland | 5,696 | 7.87 | 7,154 | 9.13 |
| Qualifications | | | | |
| Other (non-degree) (base) | 45,613 | 63.05 | 50,308 | 64.23 |
| Degree | 10,501 | 14.52 | 10,353 | 13.22 |
| No qualifications | 16,223 | 22.43 | 17,663 | 22.55 |
| Social class | | | | |
| Non-manual (base) | 48,444 | 66.97 | 62,998 | 80.43 |
| Manual | 23,893 | 33.03 | 15,326 | 19.57 |

heterogeneity. Controlling for individual-specific and time-invariant heterogeneity leads the coefficients on the regional, manual, and marital status variables to become not statistically significant because there is little within-respondent variation in these variables. Having controlled for several potential sources of bias in the causal relationship between depression and claiming DBs, we find a significantly reduced effect, 12.5 to 0.5 percentage points for males, and 8.0 to 0.7 percentage points for females.

To test whether the effects of depression are robust to alternative specifications we conduct several robustness checks. Table 6 contains the key results from the models estimated over the shorter period (1998–2007) including area wage (logged) and unemployment rates, results where GHQ caseness is used as a measure of mental health rather than depression, and results from estimation using only the balanced sample.

The first panel of results in table 6 contains the results from the final models of tables 4 and 5. The second panel of results are for the models estimated on the smaller sample but excluding the area rates. This was performed to ensure the differences in the estimates when including area rates were not due to a change in the sample. The third panel of results are where the area rates are included. When including aggregate LAD variables the sample is restricted to waves 8–17 (1998–2007). This reduces the sample to 83,559 person-year observations (40,286 male observations and 43,273 female observations) and 14,847 individuals

Table 4

Regression models for whether individual claims Disability Benefits in the next period – males

| | Pooled | Pooled with covariates | Random-effects | Random-effects dynamic | Random-effects dynamic and time averages |
|---|---|---|---|---|---|
| Depressed | 0.1249** (0.0026) | 0.0659** (0.0021) | 0.0139** (0.0013) | 0.0158** (0.0016) | 0.0047** (0.0017) |
| DB claim in past year | | | | 0.0444** (0.0026) | 0.0444** (0.0023) |
| DB claim in first year | | | | 0.0358** (0.0018) | 0.0263* (0.0019) |
| Ethnic minority | | −0.0065 (0.0038) | −0.0031 (0.0024) | −0.0020 (0.0026) | −0.0031 (0.0028) |
| Recall period (days) | | −0.0001** (0.0000) | 0.0000 (0.0000) | 0.0000 (0.0000) | 0.0000 (0.0000) |
| Education (base other) | | | | | |
| No qualifications | | 0.0132** (0.0016) | 0.0071** (0.0013) | 0.0050** (0.0013) | −0.0097 (0.0078) |
| Degree | | −0.0409** (0.0038) | −0.0153** (0.0026) | −0.0156** (0.0027) | −0.0024 (0.0080) |
| Age (base 16–20) | | | | | |
| 21–25 | | 0.0232** (0.0051) | 0.0093* (0.0021) | 0.0074** (0.0028) | 0.0077* (0.0035) |
| 26–30 | | 0.0294** (0.0050) | 0.0152** (0.0023) | 0.0109** (0.0029) | 0.0142** (0.0044) |
| 31–35 | | 0.0347** (0.0048) | 0.0155** (0.0024) | 0.0101** (0.0029) | 0.0130* (0.0052) |
| 36–40 | | 0.0393** (0.0048) | 0.0181** (0.0025) | 0.0134** (0.0030) | 0.0187** (0.0059) |
| 41–45 | | 0.0430** (0.0048) | 0.0206** (0.0027) | 0.0156** (0.0030) | 0.0225** (0.0066) |
| 46–50 | | 0.0549** (0.0048) | 0.0264** (0.0029) | 0.0199** (0.0031) | 0.0294** (0.0074) |
| 51–55 | | 0.0615** (0.0049) | 0.0302** (0.0031) | 0.0230** (0.0032) | 0.0358** (0.0081) |
| 56–59 | | 0.0707** (0.0050) | 0.0350** (0.0034) | 0.0260** (0.0033) | 0.0408** (0.0088) |
| 60–64 | | 0.0713** (0.0051) | 0.0349** (0.0034) | 0.0215** (0.0033) | 0.0493** (0.0095) |
| Health problems | | | | | |
| Arms or legs | | 0.0511** (0.0015) | 0.0117** (0.0011) | 0.0138** (0.0012) | 0.0044* (0.0013) |
| Sight | | 0.0192** (0.0030) | 0.0033** (0.0013) | 0.0040* (0.0020) | 0.0007 (0.0023) |
| Hearing | | 0.0032 (0.0023) | 0.0018 (0.0011) | 0.0028 (0.0016) | 0.0010 (0.0021) |
| Skin | | −0.0044 (0.0025) | −0.0010 (0.0012) | −0.0018 (0.0017) | −0.0004 (0.0021) |
| Chest, breathing | | 0.0181** (0.0019) | 0.0048** (0.0010) | 0.0047** (0.0013) | 0.0014 (0.0018) |

| | (1) | (2) | (3) | (4) |
|---|---|---|---|---|
| Heart and blood | 0.0346** (0.0019) | 0.0073** (0.0010) | 0.0075** (0.0013) | 0.0002 (0.0017) |
| Stomach, liver, kidney | 0.0249** (0.0022) | 0.0063** (0.0011) | 0.0071** (0.0015) | 0.0018 (0.0018) |
| Diabetes | 0.0186** (0.0033) | 0.0048* (0.0019) | 0.0045 (0.0025) | −0.0097* (0.0040) |
| Epilepsy | 0.0539** (0.0057) | 0.0117** (0.0035) | 0.0094* (0.0045) | −0.0054 (0.0074) |
| Migraine | 0.0156** (0.0028) | 0.0061** (0.0013) | 0.0067** (0.0019) | 0.0055* (0.0023) |
| Other | 0.0520** (0.0029) | 0.0106** (0.0014) | 0.0144** (0.0020) | 0.0064** (0.0021) |
| **Region (base London)** | | | | |
| South East | −0.0019 (0.0042) | 0.0003 (0.0029) | −0.0012 (0.0032) | −0.0050 (0.0088) |
| South West | 0.0039 (0.0047) | 0.0030 (0.0034) | 0.0006 (0.0036) | 0.0031 (0.0123) |
| East Anglia | 0.0079 (0.0057) | 0.0057 (0.0038) | 0.0025 (0.0044) | 0.0171 (0.0111) |
| East Midlands | 0.0259** (0.0043) | 0.0101** (0.0032) | 0.0094** (0.0034) | −0.0004 (0.0121) |
| West Midlands | 0.0203** (0.0045) | 0.0095** (0.0033) | 0.0068 (0.0035) | 0.0157 (0.0156) |
| North West | 0.0312** (0.0042) | 0.0135** (0.0032) | 0.0089** (0.0033) | 0.0175 (0.0130) |
| Yorks. & Humber. | 0.0225** (0.0044) | 0.0128** (0.0032) | 0.0102** (0.0034) | 0.0128 (0.0132) |
| North East | 0.0452** (0.0044) | 0.0207** (0.0035) | 0.0171** (0.0035) | 0.0171 (0.0142) |
| Wales | 0.0395** (0.0040) | 0.0167** (0.0030) | 0.0119** (0.0031) | 0.0075 (0.0136) |
| Scotland | 0.0291** (0.0040) | 0.0110** (0.0029) | 0.0085** (0.0031) | 0.0174 (0.0170) |
| Northern Ireland | 0.0467** (0.0044) | 0.0165** (0.0031) | 0.0141** (0.0033) | 0.0171 (0.0037) |
| **Marital status (base married)** | | | | |
| Couple | 0.0070** (0.0026) | 0.0028* (0.0014) | 0.0037* (0.0018) | 0.0002 (0.0028) |
| Widowed | −0.0065 (0.0063) | 0.0028 (0.0033) | −0.0005 (0.0045) | 0.0035 (0.0070) |
| Divorced | 0.0214** (0.0029) | 0.0058** (0.0018) | 0.0056* (0.0023) | −0.0019 (0.0039) |
| Single | 0.0216** (0.0023) | 0.0070** (0.0014) | 0.0069** (0.0017) | 0.0055 (0.0032) |
| **Year (base 2007)** | | | | |
| 1991 | 0.0340** (0.0045) | 0.0105** (0.0019) | 0.0122** (0.0027) | 0.0126** (0.0037) |
| 1992 | 0.0342** (0.0045) | 0.0111** (0.0019) | 0.0131** (0.0027) | 0.0136** (0.0037) |
| 1993 | 0.0335** (0.0046) | 0.0100** (0.0019) | 0.0106** (0.0028) | 0.0109** (0.0036) |
| 1994 | 0.0380** (0.0045) | 0.0122** (0.0019) | 0.0151** (0.0027) | 0.0153* (0.0035) |
| 1995 | 0.0303** (0.0047) | 0.0086** (0.0019) | 0.0079** (0.0028) | 0.0077* (0.0035) |
| 1996 | 0.0210** (0.0047) | 0.0064** (0.0018) | 0.0069* (0.0028) | 0.0073* (0.0034) |

(continued)

Table 4

(*Continued*)

| | Pooled | Pooled with covariates | Random-effects | Random-effects dynamic | Random-effects dynamic and time averages |
|---|---|---|---|---|---|
| **Year (base 2007) (cont.)** | | | | | |
| 1997 | | 0.0213** (0.0045) | 0.0057** (0.0018) | 0.0047 (0.0027) | 0.0050 (0.0032) |
| 1998 | | 0.0203** (0.0045) | 0.0052** (0.0018) | 0.0052 (0.0027) | 0.0053 (0.0031) |
| 1999 | | 0.0284** (0.0041) | 0.0086** (0.0017) | 0.0104** (0.0025) | 0.0103** (0.0028) |
| 2000 | | 0.0180** (0.0043) | 0.0042* (0.0017) | 0.0028 (0.0026) | 0.0027 (0.0029) |
| 2001 | | 0.0106** (0.0041) | 0.0024 (0.0015) | 0.0022 (0.0024) | 0.0025 (0.0027) |
| 2002 | | 0.0093* (0.0041) | 0.0025 (0.0015) | 0.0036 (0.0024) | 0.0041 (0.0027) |
| 2003 | | 0.0090* (0.0041) | 0.0030* (0.0015) | 0.0046 (0.0024) | 0.0055* (0.0026) |
| 2004 | | 0.0035 (0.0043) | 0.0007 (0.0016) | -0.0004 (0.0025) | -0.0003 (0.0027) |
| 2005 | | 0.0019 (0.0043) | 0.0001 (0.0016) | 0.0003 (0.0025) | 0.0004 (0.0026) |
| 2006 | | 0.0011 (0.0043) | 0.0004 (0.0016) | 0.0020 (0.0025) | 0.0025 (0.0025) |
| **Kids (base none)** | | | | | |
| 1 | | -0.0006 (0.0023) | -0.0012 (0.0010) | -0.0011 (0.0015) | -0.0026 (0.0019) |
| 2 | | 0.0020 (0.0026) | -0.0013 (0.0012) | -0.0004 (0.0017) | -0.0039 (0.0024) |
| 3+ | | 0.0129** (0.0034) | 0.0016 (0.0017) | 0.0027 (0.0023) | -0.0035 (0.0033) |
| Manual class | | 0.0325** (0.0016) | 0.0165** (0.0016) | 0.0136** (0.0013) | -0.0151 (0.0247) |
| Average depression | | | | | 0.0358** (0.0033) |
| Observations | 72,337 | 72,337 | 72,337 | 72,337 | 72,337 |
| Rho | | | 0.6952** (0.0124) | 0.476** (0.0203) | 0.3292** (0.0206) |
| Log likelihood | -14082.892 | -10222.572 | -7744.7929 | -6745.2979 | -6477.7961 |

*Notes:* standard errors in parentheses; * p-value < 0.05; ** p-value < 0.01; average marginal effects; time averages of all other covariates included in model (5) but not reported; null hypothesis of joint insignificance of the averages rejected for model (5) with p-value < 0.0001.

## Table 5

Regression models for whether individual claims Disability Benefits in the next period – females

| | Pooled | Pooled with covariates | Random-effects | Random-effects dynamic | Random-effects dynamic and time averages |
|---|---|---|---|---|---|
| Depressed | 0.0801** (0.0018) | 0.0486** (0.0015) | 0.0069** (0.0008) | 0.0121** (0.0010) | 0.0070** (0.0012) |
| DB claim in past year | | | | 0.0310** (0.0022) | 0.0326** (0.0021) |
| DB claim in first year | | | | 0.0287** (0.0015) | 0.0268** (0.0016) |
| Ethnic minority | | 0.0046 (0.0031) | 0.0003 (0.0011) | 0.0018 (0.0019) | 0.0011 (0.0021) |
| Recall period (days) | | −0.0001** (0.0000) | 0.0000* (0.0000) | 0.0000* (0.0000) | 0.0000 (0.0000) |
| Education (base other) | | | | | |
| No qualifications | | 0.0093** (0.0016) | 0.0018** (0.0006) | 0.0028* (0.0011) | −0.0107 (0.0059) |
| Degree | | −0.0133** (0.0025) | −0.0037** (0.0009) | −0.0049** (0.0016) | −0.0048 (0.0043) |
| Age (base 16–20) | | | | | |
| 21–25 | | 0.0126** (0.0048) | 0.0038** (0.0011) | 0.0040 (0.0022) | 0.0039 (0.0029) |
| 26–30 | | 0.0230** (0.0045) | 0.0059** (0.0012) | 0.0066** (0.0022) | 0.0056 (0.0036) |
| 31–35 | | 0.0280** (0.0045) | 0.0061** (0.0012) | 0.0076** (0.0023) | 0.0053 (0.0041) |
| 36–40 | | 0.0351** (0.0044) | 0.0075** (0.0013) | 0.0093** (0.0022) | 0.0079 (0.0046) |
| 41–45 | | 0.0379** (0.0044) | 0.0081** (0.0013) | 0.0093** (0.0023) | 0.0093 (0.0052) |
| 46–50 | | 0.0394** (0.0044) | 0.0092** (0.0014) | 0.0105** (0.0023) | 0.0114* (0.0057) |
| 51–55 | | 0.0446** (0.0045) | 0.0110** (0.0015) | 0.0119** (0.0024) | 0.0141* (0.0063) |
| 56–59 | | 0.0359** (0.0046) | 0.0097** (0.0015) | 0.0061* (0.0025) | 0.0098 (0.0069) |
| Health problems | | | | | |
| Arms or legs | | 0.0419** (0.0014) | 0.0051** (0.0006) | 0.0095** (0.0009) | 0.0029** (0.0011) |
| Sight | | 0.0035 (0.0027) | 0.0011 (0.0006) | 0.0019 (0.0015) | 0.0022 (0.0018) |
| Hearing | | 0.0010 (0.0028) | 0.0005 (0.0007) | 0.0002 (0.0017) | −0.0002 (0.0023) |
| Skin | | −0.0037* (0.0018) | −0.0002 (0.0004) | −0.0013 (0.0010) | −0.0010 (0.0014) |
| Chest, breathing | | 0.0139** (0.0017) | 0.0027** (0.0005) | 0.0047** (0.0010) | 0.0031* (0.0015) |

(continued)

Table 5

(Continued)

| | Pooled | Pooled with covariates | Random-effects | Random-effects dynamic | Random-effects dynamic and time averages |
|---|---|---|---|---|---|
| Health problems (cont.) | | | | | |
| Heart and blood | | 0.0097** (0.0018) | 0.0018** (0.0005) | 0.0033** (0.0010) | 0.0018 (0.0014) |
| Stomach, liver, kidney | | 0.0158** (0.0019) | 0.0023** (0.0005) | 0.0037** (0.0011) | 0.0015 (0.0014) |
| Diabetes | | 0.0167** (0.0035) | 0.0030** (0.0011) | 0.0068** (0.0022) | 0.0025 (0.0036) |
| Epilepsy | | 0.0067 (0.0051) | 0.0051** (0.0015) | 0.0053 (0.0031) | 0.0069 (0.0055) |
| Migraine | | 0.0004 (0.0017) | −0.0004 (0.0004) | −0.0006 (0.0010) | −0.0012 (0.0013) |
| Other | | 0.0287** (0.0021) | 0.0039** (0.0006) | 0.0078** (0.0012) | 0.0049** (0.0013) |
| Region (base London) | | | | | |
| South East | | −0.0065 (0.0038) | −0.0004 (0.0014) | −0.0010 (0.0025) | −0.0082 (0.0065) |
| South West | | −0.0048 (0.0045) | 0.0007 (0.0016) | 0.0027 (0.0028) | −0.0022 (0.0086) |
| East Anglia | | 0.0025 (0.0055) | 0.0012 (0.0020) | 0.0040 (0.0035) | −0.0074 (0.0101) |
| East Midlands | | 0.0071 (0.0042) | 0.0030 (0.0016) | 0.0060* (0.0028) | 0.0024 (0.0093) |
| West Midlands | | 0.0141** (0.0039) | 0.0030 (0.0016) | 0.0046 (0.0027) | −0.0043 (0.0103) |
| North West | | 0.0306** (0.0037) | 0.0069** (0.0015) | 0.0111** (0.0026) | 0.0045 (0.0089) |
| Yorks. & Humber. | | 0.0013 (0.0041) | 0.0021 (0.0016) | 0.0035 (0.0027) | −0.0052 (0.0102) |
| North East | | 0.0364** (0.0039) | 0.0092** (0.0018) | 0.0128** (0.0028) | 0.0114 (0.0124) |
| Wales | | 0.0326** (0.0035) | 0.0076** (0.0015) | 0.0112** (0.0024) | 0.0064 (0.0096) |
| Scotland | | 0.0286** (0.0034) | 0.0057** (0.0014) | 0.0093** (0.0024) | 0.0049 (0.0102) |
| Northern Ireland | | 0.0406** (0.0038) | 0.0084** (0.0016) | 0.0120** (0.0025) | −0.0006 (0.0816) |
| Marital status (base married) | | | | | |
| Couple | | 0.0064** (0.0022) | 0.0002 (0.0006) | 0.0002 (0.0013) | −0.0036 (0.0020) |
| Widowed | | −0.0081 (0.0043) | −0.0024* (0.0012) | −0.0054* (0.0027) | −0.0065 (0.0042) |
| Divorced | | 0.0123** (0.0020) | 0.0022** (0.0007) | 0.0043** (0.0013) | −0.0003 (0.0023) |
| Single | | 0.0035 (0.0020) | 0.0003 (0.0006) | 0.0004 (0.0012) | −0.0034 (0.0021) |

| Year (base 2007) | (1) | (2) | (3) | (4) | (5) |
|---|---|---|---|---|---|
| 1991 | 0.0138** (0.0041) | 0.0026** (0.0009) | 0.0047* (0.0021) | 0.0038 (0.0030) | |
| 1992 | 0.0122** (0.0041) | 0.0023* (0.0009) | 0.0046* (0.0021) | 0.0039 (0.0030) | |
| 1993 | 0.0084* (0.0042) | 0.0015 (0.0009) | 0.0025 (0.0021) | 0.0017 (0.0029) | |
| 1994 | 0.0117** (0.0041) | 0.0022* (0.0009) | 0.0044* (0.0021) | 0.0039 (0.0028) | |
| 1995 | 0.0067 (0.0043) | 0.0010 (0.0009) | 0.0016 (0.0022) | 0.0009 (0.0028) | |
| 1996 | 0.0053 (0.0042) | 0.0013 (0.0009) | 0.0028 (0.0021) | 0.0024 (0.0027) | |
| 1997 | 0.0017 (0.0040) | 0.0003 (0.0008) | 0.0004 (0.0020) | -0.0002 (0.0025) | |
| 1998 | 0.0041 (0.0040) | 0.0009 (0.0008) | 0.0027 (0.0020) | 0.0024 (0.0024) | |
| 1999 | 0.0095** (0.0035) | 0.0016* (0.0007) | 0.0033 (0.0018) | 0.0031 (0.0022) | |
| 2000 | 0.0076* (0.0036) | 0.0010 (0.0007) | 0.0023 (0.0018) | 0.0020 (0.0022) | |
| 2001 | 0.0062 (0.0034) | 0.0011 (0.0007) | 0.0019 (0.0017) | 0.0020 (0.0020) | |
| 2002 | 0.0040 (0.0034) | 0.0005 (0.0007) | 0.0008 (0.0017) | 0.0010 (0.0020) | |
| 2003 | 0.0057 (0.0034) | 0.0011 (0.0007) | 0.0028 (0.0017) | 0.0031 (0.0019) | |
| 2004 | 0.0037 (0.0034) | 0.0006 (0.0007) | 0.0009 (0.0017) | 0.0011 (0.0019) | |
| 2005 | 0.0049 (0.0034) | 0.0010 (0.0007) | 0.0022 (0.0017) | 0.0023 (0.0019) | |
| 2006 | 0.0040 (0.0035) | 0.0007 (0.0007) | 0.0019 (0.0017) | 0.0022 (0.0019) | |
| Kids (base none) | | | | | |
| 1 | -0.0099** (0.0018) | -0.0016** (0.0005) | -0.0032** (0.0010) | -0.0034* (0.0013) | |
| 2 | -0.0143** (0.0022) | -0.0027** (0.0006) | -0.0065** (0.0013) | -0.0067** (0.0018) | |
| 3+ | -0.0213** (0.0033) | -0.0045** (0.0010) | -0.0096** (0.0019) | -0.0121* (0.0027) | |
| Manual class | 0.0143** (0.0015) | 0.0045** (0.0007) | 0.0054** (0.0011) | 0.0049 (0.0178) | |
| Average depression | | | | | 0.0168** (0.0022) |
| Observations | 78,324 | 78,324 | 78,324 | 78,324 | 72,337 |
| Rho | | 0.7170** (0.0114) | 0.3937** (0.0214) | 0.3945** (0.0223) | |
| Log likelihood | -11938.305 | -9803.684 | -6918.587 | -6122.894 | -5981.394 |

*Notes:* * p-value < 0.05; ** p-value < 0.01; standard errors in parentheses; average marginal effects; time averages of all other covariates included in model (5) but not reported; null hypothesis of joint insignificance of the averages rejected for model (5) with p-value < 0.0001.

Table 6

Regression models containing area wage and unemployment effects; balanced sample estimates; and General Health Questionnaire caseness estimates

| | Final model | Area specification sample excluding area rates | Area specification sample with area wage and unemployment rates | GHQ caseness as measure for depression sample | GHQ caseness as measure for depression | Balanced sample |
|---|---|---|---|---|---|---|
| **Males** | | | | | | |
| Depressed GHQ Caseness | 0.0047** (0.0017) | 0.0021 (0.0022) | 0.0021 (0.0022) | 0.0043* (0.0018) | | 0.0051 (0.0031) |
| Area unemp. rate | | | 0.0017** (0.0006) | | 0.0048** (0.0012) | |
| Area wage rate | | | 0.0042 (0.0079) | | | |
| Observations | 72,337 | 40,286 | 40,286 | 70,615 | 70,615 | 24,817 |
| **Females** | | | | | | |
| Depressed GHQ Caseness | 0.0070** (0.0012) | 0.0068** (0.0016) | 0.0068** (0.0016) | 0.0068** (0.0012) | | 0.0050** (0.0019) |
| Area unemp. rate | | | 0.0012* (0.0005) | | 0.0064** (0.0009) | |
| Area wage rate | | | 0.0079 (0.0069) | | | |
| Observations | 78,324 | 43,273 | 43,273 | 76,623 | 76,623 | 28,801 |

*Notes:* * p-value < 0.05; ** p-value < 0.01; random-effects dynamic probit models; in addition to the area rates, the same covariates are included as those in the final models of tables 4 and 5 but not reported; standard errors in parentheses; average marginal effects; sample size for the GHQ caseness specification differs to the main estimation sample due to non-response in the GHQ; the balanced sample is the sample of individuals present in each wave of the BHPS; null hypothesis of joint insignificance of the averages rejected for all models with p-values < 0.0001.

(7,222 men, 7,625 women). The effect of depression is reduced further to an insignificant 0.2 percentage points for males, but the second panel of results reveal that this decline is due to the change in the sample. For females the effect of depression is constant across all three models at approximately 0.7 percentage points. While we find no evidence of a significant effect of local wages, we find a positive effect of the unemployment rate on the probability of claiming DBs for males and females.

Our interest lies in the effect of depression on the probability of claiming DBs in the following year. To test whether our results were sensitive to the measure of depression used, table 6 gives the key results where we model depression using a binary variable for GHQ caseness. We find a similar impact of GHQ caseness on the probability of claiming DBs as that found for the depression measure (for males 0.43 percentage points for depression [females, 0.68] and 0.48 percentage points for GHQ caseness [females, 0.64]).

Our final robustness check is with regards to attrition. If attrition is correlated with claiming DBs and/or depression our results could be biased. In the balanced panel we find no significant effect of depression on claiming DBs for males. For females, depression increased the probability of claiming DBs by 0.5 percentage points (0.2 percentage points lower than the unbalanced panel). Although attrition is an issue of statistical precision for males, the estimated effect of 0.0047 in the final model compared to 0.0051 in the balanced sample is economically equivalent. For females attrition appears not to be an issue as both the significance and size of the effect of depression are approximately equivalent in both the final model sample and the balanced sample.

## Discussion

We find a positive association between depression and the probability of claiming DBs but this effect is reduced, though remains statistically significant and positive, when we control for a number of other factors.

Making the model dynamic effectively permits past depression to affect the probability of claiming DBs. The total effect of depression thus comprises of an immediate effect, or short-run elasticity; given by the estimated coefficient for depression; an average effect, and a long-run effect which is the product of recursive effects of past depression (captured in the lagged claiming DBs effect). Given the estimates for lagged claiming DBs for males and females in our preferred specifications are small (0.0444 and 0.0326), the long-run effect is likely to be small – for example, a one period lagged impact of depression would be 0.00021 ($= \hat{\beta}_3 * \hat{\beta}_1 = 0.0444 * 0.0047$) for males and 0.00023 ($= 0.0326 * 0.0070$) for females.

Although the estimates on average depression (0.0358 and 0.0168 for males and females, respectively) are greater in magnitude than the short-run effect (0.0047 and 0.0067) inference cannot be made on the average effect due to our assumption that this signifies correlation between time-invariant depression and time-invariant individual unobserved heterogeneity (see equation (2)). However, an alternative way of interpreting the current depression and average-depression estimates is in a temporal setting. The current depression indicator measures the impact of changes in depression, while the average-depression measure picks up a longer-term propensity to depression. Hauk and Rice (2004) find significant mobility in mental health in the BHPS using the GHQ score suggesting there is enough variation to distinguish between these effects.

Comparing across the health conditions, depression had the highest effect on the probability of claiming DBs over all other conditions listed for females. For males, however, the effects of diabetes, migraine, and other conditions were larger. There are large and significant effects of those other health problems in most models. This suggests there would be significant confounding were we to exclude these other problems.

We find an increasing probability of claiming DBs by age group for both genders. Similar age effects have been found in Molho (1989, 1991) for on-flows, Lynch (1991) and Holmes and Lynch (1990) for reduced off-flows, and Disney and Webb (1991) and Beatty et al. (2009, 2010, 2013) for claiming DBs.

We find no significant effect of area wage rates for either gender, which contrasts with positive effects for on-flows to DBs for income and rate of benefit found in Molho (1989) and negative effects of DB rates on off-flows in Holmes and Lynch (1990) and positive effects of replacement rates on claiming DBs in Disney and Webb (1991). However, our results show a significant effect of higher unemployment rates on the probability of claiming DBs for males, providing support for the hidden unemployment theory. Positive effects of local unemployment rates have been found by Beatty et al. (2000) and Disney and Webb (1991), and negative effects for off-flows (Lynch 1991; Holmes and Lynch 1990). Insignificant unemployment rates were found in studies for DB on-flows by Molho (1989, 1991).

There are a number of limitations to our analyses. First, the health problems are self-reported rather than clinically diagnosed. Claiming DBs may encourage individuals to report more health problems to justify their economic situation, though our use of health information prior to claiming DBs mitigate this problem. Second, the timing of the DB claim is retrospective meaning we cannot infer whether the reported health problem was present at the time of the claim. Modelling of claiming DBs in the next period may mitigate this effect, but there may still be room for error. Third, attrition is likely to be higher amongst individuals with poor health – this has been confirmed in Contoyannis et al. (2004) who use the BHPS to analyze health dynamics. This could lead to negative bias on the effect of depression if those leaving the sample were also more likely to claim DBs. Attrition however, was found to have an insignificant impact on the estimated determinants of self-reported health in Contoyannis et al. (2004). Our results suggest that while attrition impacts on the statistical significance of the depression estimate (for males), the economic significance remains similar to the unbalanced sample (approximately 0.5 percentage points for males and females in both samples).

Our results suggest that univariate cross-sectional associations between health and claiming DBs are substantially inaccurate estimates of the causal effect of health problems on benefit claiming. For example, the estimated effects of becoming depressed on the probability of claiming DBs drop to just 0.5 and 0.7 percentage points, for males and females, respectively. These results have significant policy implications. It is unlikely that the removal of a health problem (or accommodation of that problem to enable individuals to be active in the labour market) would have the effect of reducing claimants by as much as is suggested by cross-sectional rates of health specific DB claiming.

Our findings suggest that health matters, but there are other factors influencing DB claiming. One potential explanation as to why health does not appear as the dominant/only factor in claiming DBs could lie in the hidden unemployment theory, whereby those struggling to find employment are moved between alternative state benefits. Under this scenario, health state plays only part of the process by which claiming DBs occurs. Our results suggest age and calendar year play some role under this mechanism for men, and age and the presence of children for women.

Our results also suggest that in addition to health state, there are other influences including considerable persistence in claiming and individual tendencies to claim (unobserved heterogeneity) on the probability of claiming DBs. Policy needs to target these determinants in addition to adopting interventions to improve the health of the working-age population. The change in work incapacity assessment from work capabilities to personal capabilities with the introduction of the ESA in 2008 may have helped target these additional influences.

Behind this analysis lies an assumption that claiming work incapacity benefits is detrimental to both the government and the individual. But the benefits of transitions from work incapacity may only be realized if met with re-employment that is effective in accommodating the individual's health needs, transitions to unemployment has been found to worsen health and well-being (Waddell and Burton 2006).

### Acknowledgements

The BHPS was made available through the ESRC Data Archive. The data were originally collected by the ESRC Research Centre on Micro-social Change at the University of Essex (now incorporated within the Institute for Social and Economic Research). Neither the original collectors of the data nor the Archive bear any responsibility for the analyses or interpretations presented here. The authors thank both organizations for providing access to the data. The comments of participants at the January 2009 Health Economists' Study Group (in particular, Nicholas Ziebarth) and the 2009 BHPS Conference are gratefully acknowledged.

# Notes

* *Conflict of interest:* neither author has any conflict of interest relating to this research, nor are there any political conflicts of interests related to this work. *JEL Classification:* C23, H51, I10, I18.
** Corresponding author.
1. We use the term 'disability benefits' (DBs) to cover claims for long-term sickness and/or disability by those of working age. In the UK this covers Invalidity Benefit and Sickness Benefit (DB claimants until 1995), Incapacity Benefit (new DB claimants from 1995 to 2008), and the current DB – Employment and Support Allowance.

# References

American Psychiatric Association (APA) (1994), *Diagnostic and Statistical Manual of the American Psychiatric Association*, 4th edn, Arlington, VA: American Psychiatric Publishing.

Bambra, C. (2011), *Work, Worklessness and the Political Economy of Health*, Oxford: Oxford University Press.

Barnes, H. and Sissons, P. (2013), Redefining fit for work: welfare reform and the introduction of the Employment Support Allowance. In C. Lindsay and D. Houston (eds), *Disability Benefits, Welfare Reform and Employment Policy*, Basingstoke: Palgrave Macmillan, pp. 72–93.

Beatty, C., Fothergill, S. and Houston, D. (2013), The impact of the UK's disability benefit reforms. In C. Lindsay and D. Houston (eds), *Disability Benefits, Welfare Reform and Employment Policy*, Basingstoke: Palgrave Macmillan, pp. 134–52.

Beatty, C., Fothergill, S. and MacMillan, R. (2000), A theory of employment, unemployment and sickness, *Regional Studies*, 34, 7: 617–30.

Beatty, C., Fothergill, S., Houston, D., Powell, R. and Sissons, P. (2009), A gendered theory of employment, unemployment and sickness, *Environment and Planning C: Government and Policy*, 27, 6: 958–74.

Beatty, C., Fothergill, S., Houston, D., Powell, R. and Sissons, P. (2010), Bringing Incapacity Benefit numbers down: to what extent do women need a different approach? *Policy Studies*, 31, 2: 143–62.

Black, C. (2008), *Working for a Healthier Tomorrow*, London: The Stationery Office.

Ceolta-Smith, J., Salway, S. and Tod, A. (2015), A review of health-related support provision within the UK Work Programme – what's on the menu? *Social Policy & Administration*, 49, 2: 254–76.

Contoyannis, P., Jones, A. M. and Rice, N. (2004), Simulation-based inference in dynamic panel probit models: an application to health, *Empirical Economics*, 29, 1: 49–77.

Costigan, P., Finch, H., Jackson, B., Legard, R. and Ritchie, J. (1999), *Overcoming Barriers: Older People and Income Support. Department of Social Security Research Report 100*, Leeds: Corporate Document Services.

Disney, R. and Webb, S. (1991), Why are there so many long term sick in Britain? *The Economic Journal*, 101: 252–62.

Faggio, G. and Nickell, S. (2005), *Inactivity Among Prime Age Men in the UK, Discussion Paper No. 673*, London: Centre for Economic Performance.

Goldberg, D. P., Gater, R., Sartorius, N. *et al.* (1997), The validity of two versions of the GHQ in the WHO study of mental illness in general health care, *Psychological Medicine*, 27, 2: 191–7.

Green, A. and Shuttleworth, I. (2013), Are incapacity benefit claimants beyond employment? Exploring issues of employability. In C. Lindsay and D. Houston (eds), *DBs, Welfare Reform and Employment Policy*, Basingstoke: Palgrave Macmillan, pp. 54–71.

Hauk, K. and Rice, N. (2004), A longitudinal analysis of mental health mobility in Britain, *Health Economics*, 13, 10: 981–1001.

Holmes, P. and Lynch, M. (1990), An analysis of Invalidity Benefit claim duration for new male claimants in 1977/1978 and 1982/1983, *Journal of Health Economics*, 9, 1: 71–83.

Kellett, S., Bickerstaff, D., Purdie, F., Dyke, A., Filer, S., Lomax, V. and Tomlinson, H. (2011), The clinical and occupational effectiveness of condition management for Incapacity Benefit recipients, *British Journal of Clinical Psychology*, 50, 2: 164–77.

Kotecha, M., Callanan, M., Arthur, S. and Creegan, C. (1999), *Older People's Attitudes to Automatic Awards of Pension Credit*, London: Department for Work and Pensions.

Lindsay, C. and Houston, D. (2011), Fit for purpose? Welfare reform and challenges for health and labour market policy in the UK, *Environment and Planning A*, 43, 3: 703–21.

Lynch, M. (1991), The duration of Invalidity Benefit claims: a proportional hazard model, *Applied Economics*, 23, 6: 1043–52.

McVicar, D. (2006), Why do disability benefit rolls vary between regions? A review of the evidence from the USA and UK, *Regional Studies*, 40, 5: 519–33.

McVicar, D. and Anyadike-Danes, M. (2008), Panel estimates of the determinants of British regional male incapacity benefits rolls 1998–2006, *Applied Economics*, 40, 1:1–15.

Macnicol, J. (2013), A History of work-disability. In C. Lindsay and D. Houston (eds), *Disability Benefits, Welfare Reform and Employment Policy*, Basingstoke: Palgrave Macmillan, pp. 33–53.

Molho, I. (1989), A disaggregate model of flows onto invalidity benefit, *Applied Economics*, 21, 2: 237–50.

Molho, I. (1991), Going onto Invalidity Benefit – a study for women, *Applied Economics*, 23, 10: 1569–77.

Nolan, M. and Fitzroy, F. (2003), *Inactivity, Sickness and Unemployment in Great Britain: Early Analysis at the Level of Local Authorities*, Mimeo: University of Hull.

NOMISWEB (2014a), *Employment and Support Allowance and Incapacity Benefit and Severe Disability Allowance data 1997–2013, Work and Pensions Longitudinal Survey*, NOMIS Official Labour Market Statistics, London: Office for National Statistics.

NOMISWEB (2014b), *Incapacity Benefit and Severe Disability Allowance data 1997–2013, Office for National Statistics 5% National Insurance*, NOMIS Official Labour Market Statistics, London: Office for National Statistics.

NOMISWEB (2014c), *Claimant Count and Annual Survey of Hours and Earnings data 1998–2007*, NOMIS Official Labour Market Statistics, London: Office for National Statistics.

Office for National Statistics (ONS) (2014a), *The Annual Survey of Hours and Earnings 1997–2007*, London: ONS.

Office for National Statistics (ONS) (2014b), *Estimates of Claimant Count 1991–2007*, London: ONS.

Purdie, F. and Kellett, S. (2015), The influence of presenting health condition on eventual return to work for individuals receiving health-related welfare benefits, *Social Policy & Administration*, 49, 2: 236–53.

Rees, J., Whitworth, A. and Carter, E. (2014), Support for all in the UK Work Programme? Differential payments, same old problem, *Social Policy & Administration*, 48, 2: 221–39.

Sly, F., Thair, T. and Risdon, A. (1999), Disability and the labour market: results from the winter 1998/9 LFS, *Labour Market Trends*, 107: 455–66.

Taylor, M. F., Brice, J., Buck, N. and Prentice-Lane, E. (2010), *British Household Panel Survey User Manual Volume A: Introduction, Technical Report and Appendices*, Colchester: University of Essex.

University of Essex (2010a), *British Household Panel Survey: Waves 1–18 1991–2009 (computer file)*, 7th edn, Colchester: Institute for Social and Economic Research, University of Essex (UK Data Archive [distributor], July, SN: 5151).

University of Essex (2010b), *British Household Panel Survey, Waves 1–18 1991–2009: Conditional Access, Local Authority Districts* (computer file), 3rd edn, Colchester, Essex: Institute for Social and Economic Research, University of Essex (UK Data Archive [distributor], July, SN: 6027).

Waddell, G. and Burton, A. K. (2006), *Is Work Good for your Health and Well-being?* London: The Stationery Office.

Webster, D., Brown, J., Macdonald, E. and Turok, I. (2013), The interaction of health, labour market conditions and long-term sickness benefit claims in a post-industrial city: a Glasgow case study. In C. Lindsay and D. Houston (eds), *Disability Benefits, Welfare Reform and Employment Policy*, Basingstoke: Palgrave Macmillan, pp. 111–33.

Wooldridge, J. (2005), Simple solutions to the initial conditions problem in dynamic, nonlinear panel data models with unobserved heterogeneity, *Journal of Applied Econometrics* 20, 1: 39–54.

World Health Organization (WHO) (1990), *International Classification of Disease*, 10th edn, Geneva: WHO.

# 6

## The Influence of Presenting Health Condition on Eventual Return to Work for Individuals Receiving Health-Related Welfare Benefits*

### Fiona Purdie and Stephen Kellett

### Introduction

The distribution of people claiming incapacity/disability benefits (DB) is notably unequally dispersed across the UK, strongly reflecting the regional issue of post-industrial restructuring (Beatty and Fothergill 2014, 2005; Bambra and Popham 2010). Add in the socio-economic impact of a national/global recession and the position of DB claimants in sparse job markets becomes increasingly tenuous (Lindsay and Dutton 2013). This places additional pressure on health care systems (Spence 2009), due to the increased numbers experiencing the physical and emotional negative impact of enforced worklessness (Richards 2009). Rising DB costs have prompted policymakers to respond (Black 2008) and this Special Issue highlights that the policy response has been characterized by stereotypically restricting access to DB support. The wide reaching needs of people claiming DB (Bambra 2011), however, requires social policy that addresses both macro (i.e. industrial strategy that recognizes and addresses regionality) and micro-level issues (i.e. change in the health of an individual). Macro actions would aim to change the causal and maintaining socio-economic context factors of DB (i.e. a 'large lever' of change), whilst intervention at the individual health level (i.e. a 'small lever' of change) would enable DB claimants to change, for example, unhelpful coping patterns. Much of this Special Issue rightfully concerns itself with identifying and addressing macro issues, whilst this research considers whether a health intervention does help DB claimants to change their approach to their lives and how they think and feel (i.e. encouraging necessary micro level change).

*New Perspectives on Health, Disability, Welfare and the Labour Market*, First Edition.
Edited by Colin Lindsay, Bent Greve, Ignazio Cabras, Nick Ellison and Stephen Kellett.
© 2015 John Wiley & Sons, Ltd. Published 2015 by John Wiley & Sons, Ltd.

When people require DB support for health-related unemployment, a complex biopsychosocial phenomenon is evident; readiness to return to work is restricted by the complex interplay of health condition, health related beliefs/attitudes and the economic-social-cultural context (Kertay and Pendergrass 2005). Clearly, being unemployed for a health reason is different to being unemployed solely due to lack of available work, with a schism in associated need. For example, the ex-steel worker claiming DB due to chronic back and hand pain with co-morbid depression faces many more hurdles in return to work, than the person who is made redundant due to market change, but who is essentially fit and well. Responses to the ex-steel worker can be characterized by either a health-first or work-first approach (Warren *et al.* 2014). 'Health-first' policy would dictate that a change in health status was the foundation stone for sustained return to work (i.e. helping the ex-steel worker manage his pain and depression more effectively prior to initiating job searches).

'Work-first' policy dictates that returning to work provides the right corrective environment for sustained health status change (i.e. putting the same worker into work and this situation itself improving his mood, fitness and pain management skills). Despite desire to work being high in DB recipients (McQuilken *et al.* 2003), finding employment represents a multifaceted task, as it demands a mixture of better symptom management, increased motivation and sustained behaviour change (Krause *et al.* 2001). Such individual change also needs to simultaneously occur in a context of locally available and appropriate work (Patrick 2012).

If employment is secured, there is good evidence in general unemployment samples that the therapeutic nature of work typically reverses the adverse health effects of unemployment (Sainsbury *et al.* 2008; Waddell and Burton 2006; Winefield *et al.* 1991; Winefield and Tiggemann 1990). However, in DB claimants the timing of the return to work and the type of work engaged in is critical to prevent brief unsustained stints in employment, that ultimately provide the context for another health relapse and failure experience (Barnes and Sissons 2013). In response to the increased volume of DB claimants that occurred in the ten years to 1995, Pathways to Work (PtW) was introduced in 2003. PtW intended to encourage employability through early intervention to prevent welfare dependency in DB claimants. A requirement of the PtW agenda was the introduction of a Condition Management Programme (CMP). CMP used a biopsychosocial approach to enhance coping and so facilitate return to work, in a 'health-first' style approach.

A range of mainly uncontrolled evidence has been produced regarding the experience and effectiveness of CMP – which have tended to focus on employment outcomes (see e.g. Dixon *et al.* 2007). As the evidence base for CMP mainly consists of uncontrolled studies, it is very difficult to state whether it is the action of CMP or other factors that creates employment outcomes. The Bambra, Whitehead and Hamilton (2005) systematic review of the effectiveness of welfare-to-work programmes noted low programme uptake, but a range of 11–50 per cent gaining employment following participation. Clayton *et al.* (2011) noted that the roles of personal advisers and individual case managers in CMP were the factors that helped DB claimants back to work, but that time pressures, lack of trust and job outcome targets slanted the work of case managers towards 'easier-to-place' DB claimants. Joyce *et al.* (2010) used a qualitative methodology with groups (N = 4) and individuals (N = 9), and found that whilst concerns were raised about the brevity/accessibility of CMP, participants did report a change to their health behaviours and sense of selves. Demou, Gibson and Macdonald (2012) found that the majority of claimants had mental health conditions and whilst there was a low CMP completion rate, completion was associated with improved mental health outcomes. Warren, Wistow and Bambra (2014) found that health improvement was less likely for older female CMP participants and those with a musculoskeletal condition, whilst service aspects had no impact. Kellett *et al.* (2013) in a large scale and longitudinal CMP evaluation found that remaining on DB eventually removed the gains in mental health and functioning accrued from initial CMP participation. Warren, Wistow and Bambra (2014) compared outcomes for claimants either receiving DB plus CMP (N = 139) or purely DB (N = 229). Health in the DB alone group was stable, whilst CMP produced positive changes in quality of life and mental health.

In conclusion, whilst many vocational rehabilitation programmes have been previously devised and delivered for DB populations, reviews find only modest evidence of effectiveness regarding return to work rates (Audhoe *et al.* 2010). In terms of evidence-based policy guidance, much less is known about the differential role that physical and mental health conditions may play in terms of receptivity to health intervention in enhancing or suppressing subsequent employability (Hayday *et al.* 2008). For example, whilst it is acknowledged (Barnes and Mercer 2005; Boardman *et al.* 2003) that physical and mental health conditions may create different impediments, Brouwer *et al.* (2010) failed to find that presenting health condition actually influenced the likelihood of return to work. Policy guidance is also hampered by programme evaluation focusing on *either* mental *or* physical health conditions (precluding condition comparisons) and tending to focus on the outcomes of 'high intensity' individual rehabilitation programmes – i.e. the provision of complex multi-modal interventions aimed at treating the specific physical or mental health condition creating unemployment (see e.g. Murphy *et al.* 2009). The current study is novel as:

1. it seeks to investigate whether DB recipients (due to the presence of physical or mental health problems) respond differently to a 'low intensity' health intervention; and
2. it seeks to examine whether extant health condition exerts an influence on return to work rates – over both the short and the long term.

The study hypotheses were as follows:

H1    physical and mental health conditions will return to work at similar rates at short and long term follow-up; and

H2    there will be no difference between physical and mental health conditions in terms of responsivity to intervention.

## Method

### Organizational context

CMPs were created in the UK as an aspect of the PtW (DWP 2002) employment policy context. CMP delivered disability management to recipients of health-related unemployment welfare, with the specific aim of increasing the employability of participants, via increased health condition management (Dorsett 2008). The range of health conditions seen in CMP were mental health, cardiovascular, musculoskeletal as well as other miscellaneous physical conditions, with mental health conditions prevailing (Barnes and Hudson 2006). All participants $(N = 3,794)$ in the sample were:

1.    unemployed;
2.    receiving DBs (Incapacity Benefit or Employment and Support Allowance welfare); and
3.    attending the publicly-funded South Yorkshire CMP.

Participants were referred to the programme by their Incapacity Benefit adviser, however, participation in CMP was entirely voluntary, consistent with the national programme protocol. Inclusion criteria for CMP participation was the presence of either a mental or a physical health condition which had impacted functioning and the receipt of current DBs at the time of referral. Participants were excluded from the group programme if they were deemed unable to make use of the group format or content of the intervention as a result of intellectual disability or the presence of a severe and enduring mental health condition (such as psychosis) which was currently acutely impacting functioning. Reasonable adjustments and individualized intervention was provided as an alternative where appropriate. The data presented in this article was routinely collected by the South Yorkshire CMP from the group programme only and therefore is a representative cohort. Relevant ethical approval for analyzing the data was attained from the Barnsley Primary Care Trust Research and Development Department.

### Intervention

The treatment programme was delivered via seven consecutive four-hour weekly sessions, facilitated by two CMP practitioners, to an average of N = 6 participants. CMP was theoretically grounded in Williams' (2006a, 2006b) 'five areas' approach to enhanced psychological well-being and included sessions, for example, on improving mood through increased activity, managing anxiety, improving sleep, healthy lifestyle and pacing. All of the mixed-condition group-based psycho-educational sessions were delivered in local community settings (e.g. leisure centres and voluntary organizations), with the aim of reducing any disabling effects of stigma and for ease of local access (Kellett *et al.* 2007).

## Design

In a longitudinal design, psychological and employment outcomes were collected at four time points:

1. prior to CMP (assessment);
2. immediately following CMP (termination);
3. at short-term follow-up (three months following CMP); and
4. at long-term follow-up (12–30 months following CMP).

## Participants

Health conditions were grouped into categories by clinical opinion and claimant report at screening for CMP (DWP 2002). Screening was conducted by CMP clinicians, who were working in a generic CMP practitioner role and were trained health professionals (e.g. occupational therapy, nursing, physiotherapy) by background. However, a formal diagnosis was not made. The four CMP categories were mental health conditions (61.7 per cent; N = 2,352, 1,083 males with a mean age of 39.95, and 1,269 females with a mean age of 39.99), musculoskeletal conditions (22.4 per cent; N = 855, 437 males with a mean age of 44.55, and 418 females with a mean age of 45.39), cardiovascular conditions (3 per cent; N = 113, 73 males with a mean age of 49.08, and 40 females with a mean age of 46.18) and miscellaneous physical conditions (13 per cent; N = 495, 248 males with a mean age of 42.40, and 247 females with a mean age of 44.10). Given the relatively lower frequencies of physical health conditions, the cardiovascular, musculoskeletal and miscellaneous physical conditions were combined into a single category, labelled 'physical condition' in subsequent analyses (38.3 per cent; N = 1,463, 758 males with a mean age of 44.28, and N = 705 females with a mean age of 44.28).

## Measures

1. The Clinical Outcomes in Routine Evaluation Outcome Measure (CORE-OM; Evans *et al.* 2002) is a measure of psychological distress which includes a cut off which signifies whether distress meets a clinical threshold (caseness). The CORE-OM has been demonstrated to have good concurrent (Evans *et al.* 2002) and discriminant validity

(Connell *et al.* 2007), sound internal and test-retest reliability (Evans *et al.* 2002) and is able to measure change (Connell *et al.* 2007). The risk scale of the CORE-OM was not used in the current study, due to the inappropriateness of the suicide and self-harm items within an occupational sample. Current sample full CORE-OM a = 0.79

2. The General Self-Efficacy Scale (GSES; Schwarzer and Jerusalem 1995) is a measure of the perception of the control that people feel they have over the content and direction of their lives. The scale has good concurrent and cross-cultural internal reliability (Schwarzer *et al.* 1997; Schwarzer and Jerusalem 1995). Current sample SES $\alpha = 0.69$

3. The Work and Social Adjustment Scale (WSAS; Mundt *et al.* 2002) is a measure of functional impairment attributable to an identified problem or condition. The WSAS has good internal and temporal reliability and is sensitive to differences in disorder severity and is able to measure change (Mundt *et al.* 2002). Current sample WSAS $\alpha = 0.69$.

*Defining outcomes*

Occupational outcome across the health conditions was a categorical measure of:

1. return to paid full or part-time work;
2. progression towards work, such as volunteering, education/training or having moved off health-related welfare either to no welfare or to non-health-related welfare; or
3. remaining on health-related welfare.

These categories have previously been used to successfully categorize employment outcomes for the health-related unemployment (Kellett *et al.* 2011; Kellett *et al.* 2013).

The CORE-OM was the primary psychological outcome measure. 'Caseness' categorizes whether participants are above or below an empirically derived cut-off score that demarcates a clinical population pre- and post-intervention. A score above 11 defined 'caseness' on the CORE-OM (Kellett *et al.* 2013, 2011) and therefore *clinical change* occurred when a participant was below the cut-off following CMP (N.B. this was counted only if they were above the cut-off before CMP). Magnitude of change was categorized using Jacobson and Truax (1991) reliable change criteria. Reliable change occurs when a participant has sufficiently psychometrically changed during an intervention that such a change is unlikely to be due to measurement error. Following the recommendations of Evans, Margison and Barkham (1998), *reliable improvement* occurred when participant's CORE-OM score improved by equal to or more than 1.96 times the $SE_{dif}$ on the CORE-OM pre- and post-CMP. Reliable and clinically significant improvement occurred when reliable improvement on the CORE-OM occurred in the context of a category shift from case to non-case at termination. This is a credible index of *recovery* in practice-based evidence (Barkham *et al.* 2012) and is labelled as such in reporting the results of the current study. The adjusted reliable change score and 'caseness' criteria for the CORE-OM were derived from analysis of the CORE-OM national database (Barkham, personal communication, cited in Kellett *et al.* 2013, 2011) containing an N in excess of 60,000.

*Analysis strategy*

The analysis was planned in three stages to investigate the trends in the longitudinal data and test the hypotheses. First, a practice-based intention to treat analysis was completed according to the Barkham *et al.* (2012) guidelines to contextualize the results. This means that restrictive sub-samples of CMP participants patients were created from the total sample entering CMP (i.e. physical versus mental health participants defined by also either being case or non-case on the CORE-OM) whose occupational and psychological outcomes were then tracked over the duration of the CMP and at two follow-up points (short- versus long-term follow-up). Second, return to work rates for the physical and mental health conditions were calculated at termination, short- and long-term follow-up and chi-square analyses tested whether specific health conditions were associated with return to work. Lastly, mean pre–post change scores and effect sizes were calculated on psychological outcomes for physical and mental health conditions and CORE-OM improvement-recovery rates reported (see 'Defining outcomes' section above). Effect sizes were graded with Cohen's (1992) power primer and defined as $d_+ = 0.20$ as a 'small' effect, $d_+ = 0.50$ as a 'moderate' effect, $d_+ = 0.80$ as a 'large' effect. Effect sizes are a common metric used across outcome measures, which quantifies the degree of the effectiveness of an intervention. Chi-squares were then again used to test whether health conditions differed in terms of their response to the group intervention.

## Results

Figure 1 details progression of mental and physical health condition participants over time through CMP, in order to contextualize the sample clinically (see 'Measures' section above) and display associated longitudinal attrition rates. Proportionally more DB participants with mental health problems were referred to CMP (61.77 per cent) than those with physical health problems (38.22 per cent). Prior to starting CMP, the mental health condition group had significantly higher levels of psychological distress (m = 23.13), then the physical health condition group (m = 20.21), as measured by the CORE-OM (t (3786) = 14.11, p < 0.001). Furthermore, 96.19 per cent of the mental health condition group met the threshold for 'caseness' (i.e. clinically significant psychological distress) in comparison to 88.12 per cent for the physical health condition sample on the CORE-OM. However, no significant differences between health condition groups were found before CMP

Figure 1

Study attrition rates by clinical caseness and health condition

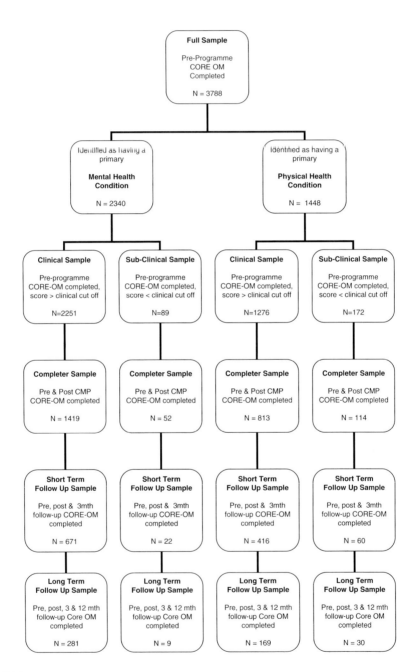

Table 1

Occupational outcome in physical and mental health conditions

|  | Termination | | Short-term follow up | | Long-term follow up | |
|---|---|---|---|---|---|---|
|  | Physical health (N = 982) | Mental health (N = 1562) | Physical health (N = 525) | Mental health (N = 720) | Physical health (N = 212) | Mental health (N = 310) |
| Return to work | 6.50% (N = 64) | 6.40% (N = 100) | 11.00% (N = 58) | 14.30% (N = 103) | 28.30% (N = 60) | 31.60% (N = 98) |
| Progress towards work | 14.40% (N = 141) | 18.80% (N = 293) | 17.30% (N = 91) | 24. 20% (N = 174) | 18.90% (N = 40) | 25.50% (N = 79) |
| Remain on benefits | 79.10% (N = 777) | 74.80% (N = 1,169) | 71.60% (N = 376) | 61.50% (N = 443) | 52.80% (N = 112) | 42.90% (N = 133) |

with regards to self-efficacy (t (4015) = −20.35, p = ns) or perceived disability (t (4019) = 0.27, p = ns). Follow-up information was attained for N = 1,169 participants at short-term (mental health condition N = 693 and physical health condition N = 476) and N = 489 participants at long-term follow-up (mental health condition health N = 290 and physical health condition N = 199).

The longitudinal return to work rates for the health condition groups are illustrated in table 1. An incremental increase in both return to work and progression towards work is evidenced across both physical and mental health conditions over time. The gap between progression and return to work rates for physical health and mental health conditions is evidenced to widen over time. This is particularly clear when reviewing the rates of participants who remained on benefits who had neither attained paid employment nor made progression towards work (such as commencing voluntary work or training). Looking at these rates specifically, the 4 per cent difference in favour of mental health conditions at termination is accordingly seen to increase to 10 per cent by both short- and long-term follow-up. Therefore there was a significant relationship between presenting health condition and employment outcome across both the short term ($\chi^2$(2, n = 939) = 9.01, p = 0.01) and long term ($\chi^2$(2, n = 520) = 7.47, p = 0.02). DB recipients with a mental health problem were significantly more likely to have made progress towards work in the short term (mental health: 24.20 per cent versus physical health: 17.30 per cent) and long term (mental health: 25.50 per cent versus physical health: 18.90 per cent) and also effectively achieved a full return to work in the short term (mental health: 14.30 per cent versus physical health: 11.00 per cent) and the long term (mental health: 31.60 per cent versus physical health: 28.30 per cent).

Table 2 reports shows the means, standard deviations (SDs) and pre–post change scores on the outcome measures, with associated effect sizes

Table 2

Clinical outcomes in health conditions

| | | Sample | Sample N | CORE-OM | | | | GSES | | | | WSAS | | | |
|---|---|---|---|---|---|---|---|---|---|---|---|---|---|---|---|
| | | | | Pre-treat. mean (SD) | Post-treat. mean (SD) | Pre-post diff. mean | Pre-post effect size (d) | Pre-treat. mean (SD) | Post-treat. mean (SD) | Pre-post diff. mean | Pre-post effect size (d) | Pre-treat. mean (SD) | Post-treat. mean (SD) | Pre-post diff. mean | Pre-post effect size (d) |
| Clinical sample | Pre-post | PHC | 813 | 21.87 (5.84) | 16.15 (7.23) | 5.77 | 0.87 | 26.60 (5.92) | 29.68 (5.43) | 8.6 | 0.54 | 25.30 (8.34) | 22.42 (9.09) | 3.18 | 0.33 |
| | | MHC | 1419 | 24.77 (5.90) | 17.85 (7.42) | 6.63 | 1.03 | 22.61 (5.92) | 27.13 (5.44) | 4.6 | 0.80 | 25.44 (8.63) | 21.38 (8.94) | 4.03 | 0.46 |
| | Short-term follow-up | PHC | 416 | 21.80 (5.95) | 16.51 (7.11) | 5.36 | 0.86 | 26.43 (5.72) | 29.84 (5.28) | 7.4 | 0.62 | 25.56 (8.33) | 22.63 (8.85) | 3.06 | 0.34 |
| | | MHC | 693 | 24.36 (5.79) | 17.87 (7.67) | 6.50 | 0.96 | 22.59 (5.81) | 27.25 (5.38) | 4.88 | 0.83 | 25.30 (8.63) | 21.03 (9.15) | 4.19 | 0.48 |
| | Long-term follow-up | PHC | 169 | 22.25 (5.82) | 17.2 (7.79) | 4.98 | 0.73 | 26.57 (5.91) | 29.00 (5.83) | 2.8 | 0.41 | 25.05 (8.89) | 23.13 (9.26) | 2.08 | 0.21 |
| | | MHC | 281 | 24.23 (6.06) | 17.91 (7.54) | 6.82 | 1.26 | 23.10 (5.97) | 27.04 (5.92) | 4.c6 | 0.66 | 25.33 (8.85) | 21.41 (8.59) | 4.20 | 0.45 |
| Full sample | Pre-post | PHC | 927 | 20.21 (7.15) | 15.17 (7.44) | 5.02 | 0.69 | 26.60 (5.98) | 29.56 (5.53) | 8.5 | 0.51 | 25.21 (8.41) | 22.40 (9.20) | 3.11 | 0.32 |
| | | MHC | 1471 | 24.13 (6.65) | 17.48 (6.41) | 6.41 | 1.02 | 22.63 (5.98) | 27.10 (5.45) | 4.80 | 0.78 | 25.29 (8.70) | 21.45 (8.90) | 3.94 | 0.44 |
| | Short-term follow-up | PHC | 476 | 20.03 (7.24) | 15.51 (4.33) | 4.62 | 0.76 | 26.45 (5.73) | 29.87 (5.29) | 7.c6 | 0.62 | 25.59 (8.35) | 22.62 (8.93) | 3.09 | 0.34 |
| | | MHC | 671 | 23.88 (6.34) | 17.54 (7.80) | 6.32 | 0.89 | 22.60 (5.81) | 27.21 (5.37) | 4.c0 | 0.82 | 25.28 (8.61) | 21.09 (9.07) | 4.18 | 0.47 |
| | Long-term follow-up | PHC | 199 | 20.14 (7.48) | 15.9 (8.04) | 4.19 | 0.55 | 26.64 (5.92) | 28.97 (5.81) | 2.8 | 0.40 | 24.97 (8.85) | 23.09 (9.26) | 2.04 | 0.21 |
| | | MHC | 290 | 23.70 (6.67) | 17.55 (7.69) | 6.06 | 0.97 | 23.16 (6.06) | 27.01 (6.05) | 4.4 | 0.64 | 25.19 (8.81) | 21.45 (8.53) | 4.14 | 0.43 |

*Notes*: PHC = physical health condition; MHC = mental health condition.

(Cohen's $d+$) for both physical and mental health condition groups. The table illustrates that psychological outcomes differed according to the measure employed across both physical and mental health conditions. The mental health condition group demonstrated greater change in terms of both psychological distress, for which there was a large effect size evidenced for the mental health condition group and a moderate to large effect size in the physical health condition group, and in terms of self-efficacy, for which there was a moderate to large effect size in the mental health condition group and a moderate effect size in the physical health condition group. There was no difference in effect size between condition groups with regards to disability, with a small effect size demonstrated across both mental and physical health condition groups.

In order to analyze change at an individual as opposed to group level, table 3 documents the CORE-OM improvement (i.e. a reliable reduction in psychological distress) and recovery (i.e. reliable and clinically significant reduction in psychological distress) rates for the physical and mental health conditions over time – where participants reported clinically significant distress on the CORE-OM at assessment. Whilst the participant rates making a reliable improvement over the intervention appeared higher in the mental health condition group, chi square analysis actually revealed no significant difference between health conditions in either the completer ($\chi^2(1, n = 2,232) = 2.32, p = ns$), short-term ($\chi^2(1, n = 1,041) = 1.57, p = ns$) or long-term follow-up ($\chi^2(1, n = 438) = 0.28, p = ns$) cohorts. In terms of recovery, however, the physical health condition participants showed a significantly higher recovery rate across completer ($\chi^2(1, n = 2,232) = 21.15, p < 0.001$) and short-term cohorts $\chi^2(1, n = 1,041) = 4.67, p < 0.05$), but not in the long-term follow-up cohort ($\chi^2(1, n = 438) = 0.48, p = ns$).

## Discussion

There was a dual focus to the current DB 'health-first' programme evaluation. First, to examine whether extant health condition exerted any influence on subsequent ability to return to work, and, second, to assess whether differing health conditions responded to the health intervention (CMP) in different ways. Contrary to our hypotheses, participants presenting with a mental health condition were found to be more likely to return to work across the short and long term, than those with physical health conditions. The degree of improvement in psychological distress, disability and self-efficacy over the course of the programme at a condition group level was higher for those participants with a mental health condition.

These results are indicative that proportionally more participants with a mental health condition were able to make use of the programme in order to improve their psychological health. This may be due to a predominant focus within the CMP group intervention on managing

Table 3

Recovery and improvement rates by health conditions

| | Recovery rates | | | | Improvement rates | | | |
| | Mental health conditions | | Physical health conditions | | Mental health conditions | | Physical health conditions | |
| Clinical sample | Recovered N | Recovered % | Recovered N | Recovered % | Improved N | Improved % | Improved N | Improved % |
|---|---|---|---|---|---|---|---|---|
| Completer | 261 | 18.4% | 217 | 26.7% | 803 | 56.6% | 433 | 53.3% |
| Short-term follow-up | 126 | 18.8% | 101 | 24.3% | 357 | 53.2% | 206 | 49.5% |
| Long-term follow-up | 36 | 12.8% | 51 | 18.2% | 145 | 51.6% | 85 | 50.3% |

psychological symptoms, be these primary or secondary to long-term unemployment. Additionally, common mental health conditions may have greater 'plasticity' in terms of potential for psychological gain and associated employment change. Indeed, reaching full recovery is not necessarily required for participants with mental health conditions to make progress towards or secure employment. Previous studies of psychological and occupational outcome following CMP have found that reliable psychological improvement (i.e. a significant psychological shift rather than reaching a benchmark of complete remission of symptoms) occurring post-CMP predicted a successful return to work (Kellett *et al.* 2013). This evidence usefully revises the previous opinion that DB recipients with mental health conditions are more 'hard to help' in facilitating a return to work (Dorsett 2008; DWP 2009).

Despite lower overall rates of improvement as compared to the mental health condition group, our results indicated that a higher proportion of participants with a physical health condition achieved recovery status during CMP, i.e. those participants with a physical condition who could make use of the programme content appear to have made greater gains in terms of reaching complete psychological recovery. This may be because the psychological issues being addressed were less chronic and/or less complex than the primary psychological difficulties manifest in the mental health condition group. There are significant potential benefits to attaining psychological recovery for those with physical health conditions and our findings suggest (in combination with the high caseness rates found at assessment) that intervention is indicated on health grounds alone in this condition group. However, in terms of complete occupational rehabilitation, people experiencing chronic physical health conditions may require additional input, such as complex multimodal medical and vocational rehabilitation to facilitate an ability to return to work (Kuoppala *et al.* 2008).

The results imply that addressing the condition management difficulties which have precipitated health-related unemployment can produce psychological benefit and can positively influence the return to work prognosis for DB recipients. This evidence would be supportive of a health-first policy approach. Programmes promoting return to work for DB recipients that ignore or neglect condition management issues, may risk disregarding or overlooking a major catalyst of employment outcome. Programme content can be pragmatically grounded in cognitive-behavioural principles (such as avoidance, coping and increasing meaningful and enjoyable activity), and these conceptual elements can be sensitively and practically adapted to formulate and intervene (Winspear 2008). As return to work is ultimately a behavioural task, advice and support regarding the behavioural management of that task seems practical.

Whilst the results implicate that a cognitive-behaviourally-based intervention aimed at condition management can be a useful catalyst to return to work for DB recipients, it is also apparent that it is not a panacea. There was a 28–30 per cent return to work rate (for physical and mental health conditions, respectively) at long-term follow-up and a further 18–25 per cent had made some progress towards work such as commencing voluntary work or training (again, for physical and mental health conditions, respectively). However, this also highlights that just under one in two DB participants had not achieve any employment-related changes by long term follow-up. Of course, lack of availability of work in the local economy may also be a significant factor affecting return to work rates (Patrick 2012). For those participants who struggled to make use of and progress using a low intensity group-format psycho-educational mixed condition approach, this raises the question of what (cost-effective) health and employment intervention would produce the necessary catalytic effect? For some, an effective return to work may possibly only be facilitated through more intensive and individualized intervention approaches (e.g. a more 'high intensity' one-to-one psycho-therapeutic approach). Further research is required to establish the factors that influence both drop-out from, and/or poor capacity to utilize, return to work interventions for DB recipients. Policy regarding return to work services for DB populations would benefit from using the evidence regarding 'stepped care' service delivery models (Bower and Gilbody 2005). This would ensure that the health and employment needs are matched to the appropriate level of return to work support, with intervention duration and intensity increasing to meet and match identified individual needs. Further 'head-to-head' outcome research is needed to contrast the clinical efficacy and economic benefits of:

1.  high versus low intensity DB rehabilitation programmes; and
2.  human capital versus 'work-first' programmes for DB recipients.

In terms of informing associated policy development, such outcome research is particularly needed in DB populations that have been receiving welfare over an extended period of time.

In terms of methodological weaknesses, the main concern was lack of random allocation to active intervention and an associated no treatment control group that employment and health outcomes could have been benchmarked against (Lilienfeld 2007; Corney and Simpson 2005). The CMP evidence base contains the single controlled study (Warren *et al.* 2014). Further DB health-first policy evaluations should consider random allocation to both 'active' (e.g. another form of credible health intervention) and passive (e.g. no intervention or waiting list) control arms in any future trials. Duration of time on DB was not recorded in the current study and this is a study weakness as benefit duration predicts a poor employment prognosis (DWP 2009, 2002; Grove 2006). Similarly, the follow-up data was collected at a single point in time for all and therefore captured participants at various lengths post-CMP completion (which varied between 12 and 30 months' post-completion as described in the methodology). Future longitudinal research would benefit from more structured follow-up. The health status of the CMP participants was not formally diagnosed and therefore there was much diagnostic uncertainty in the sample. Collapsing of various health conditions into two categories (mental and physical health conditions) created broad 'catch-all' categories, which is open to criticism. The design prohibited analyzing whether it was the specific 'change methods' of CMP or simply regular participation with groups of people in a similar situation that facilitated outcomes (Vinokur and Schul 1997). A longer follow-up period would also more truly test the durability of the low intensity rehabilitation offered.

In summary, the current study investigated the impact of extant health condition on the effectiveness of a health intervention and on eventual return to work rates in a naturalistic longitudinal design with DB recipients in order to test the effectiveness of a health-first policy approach. It was found that there were differences at assessment between the health conditions, with mental health recipients reporting greater psychological distress. The longitudinal evidence highlighted that, at an individual level, mental health recipients retuned to work at higher rates over time. In terms of psychological outcomes, welfare recipients with both mental and physical health conditions benefitted. Programme participants with mental health conditions reported a greater degree of psychological change over the course of the intervention. Whilst participants with a physical health condition were most likely to make a complete psychological recovery. This evidence would suggest that 'small lever' condition management change at the level of the individual is an important component of effective return to work. Our results also suggest that future health-first provision may benefit from incorporating a 'stepped care' model of occupational rehabilitation, whereby group-based, psycho-educational condition management is provided as one of a number of interventions tailored to the degree of presenting need and complexity. We would suggest that other useful interventions would include 'higher intensity' individual psychological intervention as well as multidisciplinary approaches to enable the needs those with more chronic or complex difficulties to be addressed.

Such change, however, cannot exist in a 'large lever' policy vacuum that ignores the convincing evidence, for example, of marked regionality to DB claim rates (Beatty and Fothergill 2014). Returning to our earlier example of the steel-worker experiencing depression and chronic pain, current evidence suggests that a health-first approach would have the best chance of helping him be 'work ready'. Given the evidence across this Special Issue, it appears unwise for policymakers to solely or disproportionately emphasize work-first approaches. Effective DB social policy must integrate and balance out both a top–down and bottom–up approach to encouraging employment, in which health change or condition management change occurs in a context of available and appropriate employment opportunities. Policymakers also need to prioritize the provision of a coordinated research strategy of high quality controlled studies that effectively assess economic and health outcomes following health intervention in the truly long-term.

## Acknowledgements

With thanks to all CMP participants and staff.

## Note

\* Correspondence concerning this article should be addressed to Dr Stephen Kellett, Department of Psychology, University of Sheffield, Sheffield S10 2TN, UK. Telephone +44 (0) 114 222 6537, fax +44 (0) 114 222 6610, email s.kellett@sheffield.ac.uk.

## References

Audhoe, S. S., Hoving, J. L., Sluiter, J. K. and Frings-Dresen, M. H. W. (2010), Vocational interventions for unemployed: effects on work participation and mental distress, *Journal of Occupational Rehabilitation*, 20: 1–13.

Bambra, C. (2011), *Work, Worklessness and the Political Economy of Health*, Oxford: Oxford University Press.

Bambra, C. and Popham, F. (2010), Worklessness and regional differences in the social gradient in general health: evidence from the 2001 English census, *Health and Place*, 16, 5: 1014–21.

Bambra, C., Whitehead, M. and Hamilton, V. (2005), Does 'welfare-to-work' work? A systematic review of the effectiveness of the UK's welfare-to-work programmes for people with a disability or chronic illness, *Social Science Medicine*, 60: 1905–18.

Barkham, M., Stiles, W. B., Connell, J. and Mellor-Clark, J. (2012), Psychological treatment outcomes in routine NHS services: What do we mean by treatment effectiveness? *Psychology and Psychotherapy: Theory, Research and Practice*, 85, 1: 1–16.

Barnes, C. and Mercer, G. (2005), Disability, work and welfare: challenging the social exclusion of disabled people, *Work Employment and Society*, 19: 527–45.

Barnes, H. and Hudson, M. (2006), *Pathways to work: Qualitative research on the condition management programme*, Department for Work and Pensions Research Report 346, Leeds: DWP Publications, Corporate Document Services.

Barnes, H. and Sissons, P. (2013), Redefining fit for work: welfare reform and the introduction of the Employment Support Allowance. In C. Lindsay and D. Houston (eds), *Disability Benefits, Welfare Reform, and Employment Policy*, Basingstoke: Palgrave Macmillan.

Beatty, C. and Fothergill, S. (2005), The diversion from 'unemployment' to 'sickness' across British regions and districts, *Regional Studies*, 39: 837–54.

Beatty, C. and Fothergill, S. (2014), The local and regional impact of the UK's welfare reforms, *Cambridge Journal of Regions, Economy and Society*, 7, 1: 63–79.

Black, C. (2008), *Working for a Healthier Tomorrow*, London: The Stationery Office.

Boardman, J., Grove, B., Perkins, R. and Shepherd, G. (2003), Work and employment for people with psychiatric disabilities, *The British Journal of Psychiatry*, 182: 467–8.

Bower, P. and Gilbody, S. (2005), Managing common mental health disorders in primary care: conceptual models and evidence base, *British Medical Journal*, 330: 839–42.

Brouwer, S., Reneman, M. F., Bültmann, U., Klink, J. J. L. and Groothoff, J. W. (2010), A prospective study of return to work across health conditions:

perceived work attitude, self-efficacy and perceived social support, *Journal of Occupational Rehabilitation*, 20: 104–12.

Clayton, S., Bambra, C., Gosling, R., Povall, S., Misso, K. and Whitehead, M. (2011), Assembling the evidence jigsaw: insights from a systematic review of UK studies of individual-focussed return to work initiatives for disabled and long-term ill people, *BMC Public Health*, 11: 170.

Cohen, J. (1992), A power primer, *Psychological Bulletin*, 112, 1: 155–9.

Connell, E., Barkham, M., Stiles, W. B., Twigg, E., Singleton, N., Evans, O. and Miles, J. (2007), Distribution of CORE-OM scores in a general population, clinical cut-off points and comparison with the CIS-R, *British Journal of Psychiatry*, 190: 69–74.

Corney, R. and Simpson, S. (2005), Thirty-six month outcome data from a trial of counselling with chronically depressed patients in a general practice setting, *Psychology and Psychotherapy: Theory, Research and Practice*, 78: 1–13.

Demou, E., Gibson, I. and Macdonald, E. B. (2012), Identification of the factors associated with outcomes in a Condition Management Programme, *BMC Public Health*, 12, 1: 927.

Department for Work and Pensions (DWP) (2002), *Pathways to Work: Helping People into Employment*, London: HMSO.

Department for Work and Pensions (DWP) (2009), *Incapacity Benefit Eligibility*, London: HMSO.

Dixon, J., Mitchell, M. and Dickens, S. (2007), *Pathways to Work: Extension to Existing Customers* (matched case study), (No 148), London: Department for Work and Pensions.

Dorsett, R. (2008), *Pathways to work for new and repeat Incapacity Benefits claimants: Evaluation synthesis report*, Department for Work and Pensions Research Report 525, Leeds: DWP Publications, Corporate Document Services.

Evans, C., Connell, M., Barkham, M., Margison, F., McGrath, G., Mellor-Clark, J. and Audin, K. (2002), Towards a standardised brief outcome measure: Psychometric properties and utility of the CORE-OM, *British Journal of Psychiatry*, 180: 51–60.

Evans, C., Margison, F. and Barkham, M. (1998), The contribution of reliable and clinically significant change methods to evidence-based mental health, *Evidence Based Mental Health*, 1: 70–2.

Grove, B. (2006), Common mental health problems in the workplace; how can the occupational physicians help? *Occupational Medicine*, 56: 291–3.

Hayday, S., Rick, J., Carroll, C., Jagger, N. and Hillage, J. (2008), *Review of the effectiveness and work effectiveness of interventions, strategies and programmes and policies to help recipients of incapacity benefits return to employment (paid and unpaid)*, Evidence Review 3, National Institute for Health and Care Excellence.

Jacobson, N. S. and Truax, P. (1991), Clinical significance: a statistical approach to defining meaningful change in psychotherapy research, *Journal of Consulting and Clinical Psychology*, 59: 12–19.

Joyce, K. E., Smith, K. E., Henderson, G., Grieg, G. and Bambra, C. (2010), Patient perspectives of Condition Management Programmes as a route to better health, well-being and employment, *Family Practice*, 27: 101–9.

Kellett, S., Bickerstaffe, D., Purdie, F., Dyke, A., Filer, S., Lomax, V. and Tomlinson, H. (2011), The clinical and occupational effectiveness of condition management for Incapacity Benefit recipients, *British Journal of Clinical Psychology*, 50: 164–77.

Kellett, S., Clarke, S. and Matthews, L. (2007), Delivering group psychoeducational CBT in Primary Care: comparing outcomes with individual CBT and individual psychodynamic interpersonal psychotherapy, *British Journal of Clinical Psychology*, 46, 2: 211–22.

Kellett, S., Purdie, F., Bickerstaff, D., Hooper, S. and Scott, S. (2013), Predicting return to work from health related welfare following low intensity cognitive behaviour therapy, *Behaviour Research and Therapy*, 51: 134–41.

Kertay, L. and Pendergrass, T. M. (2005), Biopsychosocial factors in claims for disability compensation: issues and recommendations. In I. Z. Schultz and R. J. Gatchel (eds), *Handbook of Complex Occupational Disability Claims: Early Risk Identification, Intervention and Prevention*, New York, NY: Kluwer Academic.

Krause, N., Frank, J. W., Dasinger, L. W., Sullivan, T. J. and Sinclair, S. J. (2001), Determinants of duration of disability and return-to-work after work-related injury and illness: challenges for future research, *American Journal of Industrial Medicine*, 40: 464–84.

Kuoppala, J., Lamminpaa, A. and Husman, P. (2008), Work health promotion, job well being and sickness absences — a systematic review and meta-analysis, *Journal of Occupational and Environmental Medicine*, 50: 1216–27.

Lilienfeld, S. O. (2007), Psychological treatments that cause harm, *Perspectives on Psychological Science*, 2: 53–70.

Lindsay, C. and Dutton, M. (2013), Promoting health pathways to employability: lessons from the UK s welfare-to-work agenda, *Policy and Politics*, 41: 183–200.

McQuilken, M., Zahniser J. H., Novak, J., Starks, R. D., Olmos, A. and Bond, G. R. (2003), The work project survey: consumer perspectives on work, *Journal of Vocational Rehabilitation*, 18: 59–68.

Mundt, J. C., Marks, I. M., Greist, J. H. and Shear, J. H. (2002), The Work and Social Adjustment Scale: a simple accurate measure of impairment in functioning, *British Journal of Psychiatry*, 180: 461–4.

Murphy, G., Middleton, J., Quirk, R., De Wolf, A. and Cameron, I. D. (2009), Prediction of employment status one year post-discharge from rehabilitation following traumatic spinal cord injury: an exploratory analysis of participation and environmental variables, *Journal of Rehabilitation Medicine*, 41: 1074–9.

Patrick, R. (2012), Work as the primary 'duty' of the responsible citizen: a critique of this work-centric approach, *People, Place and Policy Online*, 6, 1: 5–15.

Richards, T. (2009), Governments must act now to prevent slide into poverty and ill health after recession (editorial), *British Medical Journal*, 339: 4087.

Sainsbury, R., Irvine, A., Aston, J., Wilson, S., Williams, C. and Sinclair, A. (2008), *Mental Health and Employment*, Department for Work and Pensions Research Summary, 513, Leeds: Corporate Document Services.

Schwarzer, R. and Jerusalem, M. (1995), Generalized self-efficacy scale. In J. Weinman, S. Wright and M.Johnston (eds), *Measures in Health Psychology: A User's Portfolio*, Windsor: NFER-Nelson, pp. 35–7.

Schwarzer, R., Born, A., Iwawaki, S. and Lee, Y.-M. (1997), The assessment of optimistic beliefs; comparison of Chinese, Indonesian, Japanese and Korean versions of the Generalised Self-Efficacy Scale, *Psychologio: An International Journal of the Psychology of the Orient*, 40: 1–13.

Spence, A. M. (2009), The financial and economic crisis and the developing world, *Journal of Policy Modelling*, 31: 502–8.

Vinokur, A. D. and Schul, Y. (1997), Mastery and inoculation against setbacks as active ingredients in the JOBS intervention for the unemployed, *Journal of Consulting and Clinical Psychology*, 65: 867–77.

Waddell, G. and Burton, K. (2006), *Is Work Good for your Health and Wellbeing?* London: The Stationery Office.

Warren, J., Bambra, C., Kasim, A., Garthwaite, K., Mason, J. and Booth, M. (2014), Prospective pilot evaluation of the effectiveness and cost utility of a 'health-first' case management service for long-term Incapacity Benefit recipients, *Journal of Public Health*, 36: 117–24.

Warren, J., Wistow, J. and Bambra, C. (2014), Applying qualitative comparative analysis (QCA) in public health: a case study of a health improvement service for long-term incapacity benefit recipients, *Journal of Public Health*, 36: 126–33.

Williams, C. (2006a), *Overcoming Anxiety: A Five Areas Approach*, London: Hodder Arnold.

Williams, C. (2006b), *Overcoming Depression and Low Mood*, 2nd edn, London: Hodder Arnold.

Winefield, A. H. and Tiggemann, M. (1990), Employment status and psychological well-being: a longitudinal study, *Journal of Applied Psychology*, 75: 455–9.

Winefield, A. H., Winefield, H. R., Tiggeman, M. and Goldney, R. D. (1991), A longitudinal study of the psychological effects of unemployment and unsatisfactory employment on young adults, *Journal of Applied Psychology*, 76: 424–31.

Winspear, D. (2008), Using CBT to improve mental health and employment outcomes for Incapacity Benefit customers: final report, *Journal of Occupational Psychology, Education and Disability*, 10: 91–104.

# 7

# *A Review of Health-related Support Provision within the UK Work Programme – What's on the Menu?*

## Jenny Ceolta-Smith, Sarah Salway and Angela Mary Tod

## Introduction

In common with other European welfare states, reducing the number of working age welfare benefits claimants with health-related needs by supporting them into paid employment has been a prominent policy focus for UK government since the late 1990s (DWP 2002). Initially, in 1998 the then New Labour Government introduced voluntary programmes to encourage Incapacity Benefit claimants to move into paid work via the New Deal for Disabled People (DWP 2002). This programme offered varied forms of support across the UK and later revised in 2001 (Stafford 2012). These interventions were delivered by organizations (private, public and voluntary) termed Job Brokers, who had been awarded contracts by Jobcentre Plus (a government agency that delivers back-to-work services for working age people in receipt of benefits) (Stafford 2012). However, these initiatives did not achieve the Government's target reduction in the number of Incapacity Benefit claimants (DWP 2002).

## Pathways to Work

In 2003, Pathways to Work (PtW) was introduced; a relatively structured programme aimed at those claiming sickness benefits which included an explicit focus on addressing health-related barriers to employment. The first seven pilot PtW programmes were led by Jobcentre Plus. By April 2008, PtW programmes were available across the UK with 60 per cent

*New Perspectives on Health, Disability, Welfare and the Labour Market*, First Edition.
Edited by Colin Lindsay, Bent Greve, Ignazio Cabras, Nick Ellison and Stephen Kellett.
© 2015 John Wiley & Sons, Ltd. Published 2015 by John Wiley & Sons, Ltd.

being delivered by private and voluntary sector organizations that were contracted by the Department for Work and Pensions (DWP). The PtW policy prescribed the 'Personal Adviser' (PA) role – a frontline worker who conducted a series of mandatory one-to-one work-focused interviews with claimants – and included provision of a health-focused intervention, referred to as the Condition Management Programme (CMP). The CMP was part of the 'Choices' menu that offered a range of voluntary support elements (Lindsay and Dutton 2012).

## Pathways to Work Condition Management Programme

The CMP was developed by a Joint DWP-Department of Health Ministerial Group and was designed for claimants with non-severe mental health, cardiovascular and musculoskeletal conditions (Randall 2012). A range of interventions commonly based on cognitive behavioural approaches were generally provided by healthcare professionals (Lindsay and Dutton 2010). These interventions aimed to help participants manage their health conditions in order to progress into work (Lindsay and Dutton 2012). The CMP was delivered either by National Health Service (NHS) organizations, working in partnership with Jobcentre Plus or by private contractors who had been awarded DWP contracts (Lindsay and Dutton 2012). Funding for the NHS-led CMPs was provided by the DWP and was not linked to any targets for claimant course completions or movement into work (Lindsay and Dutton 2010).

Following the expansion of the PtW programme, the responsibility for the design and delivery of CMPs moved away from the NHS. This move encouraged further heterogeneity of CMPs under the DWP's 'black box' commissioning approach which allowed contracted providers to deliver PtW and fund a CMP within this. Many of these non-NHS-led CMP interventions could be selected at the discretion of the provider. However, there was a requirement to consider the three groups of health conditions described above, local Incapacity Benefit claimant population needs, gaps in existing provision and adhere to NHS clinical governance standards (Jobcentre Plus 2006).

There have been mixed reports concerning the original aims and contribution of CMP, particularly regarding job outcomes (see Lindsay and Dutton 2013; Beatty *et al.* 2013). The DWP's commissioned PtW evaluations and other empirical research have highlighted a number of benefits and drawbacks of the CMP (Lindsay and Dutton 2013). Overall, the CMPs were found to support improvements in participants' self-reported health (Kellett *et al.* 2011). Additionally, two key CMP benefits that related to PAs' practice were:

1.  being assisted by CMP practitioners to help claimants who had complex health issues (Barnes and Hudson 2006; Nice and Davidson 2010); and
2.  improved interactions with claimants during work-focused interviews (Dickens *et al.* 2004).

However, CMP was found to be limited in a number of ways, for instance, in not fully supporting some claimants with physical health conditions nor in offering longer-term support (Lindsay and Dutton 2013). Some of the identified gaps in the PtW CMPs delivery appear to have been considered by the then Labour Government as shown in its final reform paper, *Building Bridges to Work: New Approaches to Tackling Long-term Worklessness* (DWP 2010a). This article set out proposals to develop a new expanded health-related support provision which would be accessible on a voluntary basis to a wider group of claimants including those who received Jobseeker's Allowance (a government benefit for working age people who are actively seeking work) (DWP 2010a). However, this proposed health-related support did not materialize following the change in government in 2010, being supplanted by proposals for the Work Programme, as described in the next section.

## Work Programme

PtW ended shortly before the Work Programme was launched by the current coalition Government in June 2011. This new single programme replaced most of the existing provision implemented under the Labour Government, and aims to meet the needs of nine claimant groups who are either longer-term unemployed or at risk of becoming so (DWP 2011a). The DWP (2011b) maintain that the Work Programme is designed to 'avoid many of the failings of previous employment programmes which were inflexible, short term, too expensive, and failed to support the hardest to reach customers' (DWP 2011b: 140).

The Work Programme is split into 18 contract package areas across the UK. Following a two-stage tendering process, the DWP awarded 40 contracts to 18 so-called 'Prime' provider organizations in April 2011 (Primes) (National Audit Office 2012) (Primes: A4e 2011; Avanta 2011; BEST 2011; CDG 2011; EOS 2011; ESG Holdings Limited 2011;G4S 2011; Ingeus UK Limited; JHP 2011; Maximus 2011; NCG 2011; Pertemps People Development Group 2011; Prospects 2011; Reed 2011; Rehab JobFit 2011; Seetec 2011; Serco 2011; Working Links 2011). The majority of these contracts were awarded to private organizations, bids having been assessed in relation to price and quality. Quality factors included, 'service delivery, resources, stakeholder engagement, and implementation' (House of Commons Work and Pensions Committee 2011a: 18). Each contract package area has at least two, but sometimes three, Primes. Primes hold the contracts with the DWP, but may deliver their interventions directly and/or via one or more sub-contracted organizations. Contracts were awarded for five years until March 2016, with an additional two years to complete delivery by 2018 (DWP 2011a).

The Work Programme marks a departure from PtW in several important respects. In particular, there has been a further shift towards so-called black box commissioning, through which contracted organizations are given far greater freedom to design and deliver their interventions (Rees *et al.* 2014). Furthermore, commentators have noted that ill-health has considerably less prominence in the Work Programme than in PtW. This raises concerns regarding the extent to which health-related obstacles to employment are adequately highlighted in current policy (Lindsay and Dutton 2013; Beatty *et al.* 2013; Warren *et al.* 2011). The importance of addressing claimants' health-related barriers to employment alongside other employability factors has also been demonstrated in evaluations of PtW and other research (Kemp and Davidson 2010; Beatty and Fothergill 2011; Black and Frost 2011; Lindsay and Dutton 2012). Given there is a lack of prescription within current contracts, important questions arise regarding whether and how support for claimants with health conditions will be provided across Work Programme areas and the implications for claimant outcomes.

This article begins to address these questions by examining how the Work Programme policy objectives have been responded to by Primes. This is achieved via an exploration of whether and how health-related support was described in the successful bid documents submitted to the DWP through the competitive tendering process for government contracts.

## Methods

This article draws on findings from a multi-method study that was guided by the Canadian National Collaborating Centre for Healthy Public Policy (NCCHPP) method for synthesizing knowledge about public policies (Morestin *et al.* 2010). The study employed an interpretive documentary analysis alongside other methods. It is the findings of this documentary analysis that are reported on here.

Documents are written records that are considered to be sources of information that, if obtainable, can be subjected to a quality appraisal and selected as evidence for analysis (Scott 1990). Prior (2008) presents a useful typology for analyzing documents that explains how documents can be studied in relation to their content or use and function. As such documents can be considered as both topics (e.g. in terms of content – by focusing on how a document came *'into being'*) and resources (e.g. in terms of use and function – by focusing on how a document is used by various actors) (Prior 2008: 825). Varied methodological approaches, quantitative and qualitative, and a range of methods can be adopted when conducting documentary analysis (Shaw *et al.* 2004). For example, a researcher may use a quantitative positivist methodology and method such as content analysis. Alternatively, a qualitative interpretative approach can be used that incorporates policy discourse and identifies themes, and is adopted in this study. The NCCHPP's analysis framework, as discussed below, was selected because it offered a flexible but systematic analytical approach. This method also permitted the selected documents to be viewed as both topics and resources. Therefore, there were opportunities to not only explore how the Work Programme delivery models had evolved, but how policy and other evidence sources were used by actors (i.e. Primes) to formulate these.

### Documentary sources

In order to understand in more detail the Work Programme policy and its underlying theory and assumptions, the first stage of our documentary analysis involved the location and exploration of key policy papers, ministerial statements and supporting documents such as the tender specification and supporting information. These documents were found through web-based searches which included the DWP and related government websites, such as the House of Commons Work and Pensions Committee.

Next we identified and accessed documents that could provide insight into how the national-level Work Programme policy was responded to by the Primes delivering interventions on the ground. The bid documents that were prepared and submitted to the DWP within this competitive tendering process, titled, *Employment Related Support Services Framework Agreement Mini Competitions for the Provision of the Work Programme,* form the primary data for the present study (DWP 2010c). These documents were retrieved from the Government's Contracts Finder website. These included all of the 18 Primes, some of which operate in more than one area. These documents described the Primes' delivery models, customer journeys and minimum service levels. Minimum service levels are set by each Prime. Websites were also searched for all of the Primes, and where available, their sub-contractor organizations to identify any supporting information that could give further insight into the planned delivery, such as job descriptions for PAs and healthcare professionals employed by these organizations.

### Review and synthesis approach

Documentary analysis has been used widely within health and social policy research and is often utilized at the early stages of policy innovation when there is little by way of other evidence to analyze. The NCCHPP's analysis framework advocates the reviewing of documents as an essential component of any policy analysis. It also highlights the importance of unearthing the underlying logic of the policy, its presumed intervention stages and associated assumptions. This process provides insights into the plausibility of the policy and highlights any areas that deserve scrutiny (Morestin *et al.* 2010). Thus, while recognizing that public documents – including the Work Programme policy papers and the Primes' bid documents examined here – can only ever present a 'partial or superficial account' (Shaw *et al.* 2004: 260), we nevertheless consider them to provide important insight into national policy and how it is being translated into organizational policy and operational plans. Following Shaw *et al.*'s lead (2004), we sought to go beyond the overt and explicit statements in the documents, to uncover both the rhetoric of the policy environment and indications of underpinning ideologies that shape the policy-into-practice process.

At the practical level, we followed the NCCHPP's recommendation by first reading and re-reading the retrieved documents several times prior to data extraction. An inclusive approach was taken when the documents were explored for any kind of reference to health. This included a wide variety of health conditions and other health-related issues such as drug addictions. Structured extraction templates were then developed on the basis of the emerging themes. Sections of text that concerned the identified dimensions were manually highlighted, coded, cut and pasted into the relevant sections in the extraction forms by the first author. It was necessary to re-read the bid documents and extract further data as new questions emerged and preliminary analyzes were challenged via a process of team reflection and validation. This process aimed to reduce researcher bias. Reading across the extraction templates allowed both the explicit elements of the bid documents to be compared and contrasted and the more implicit elements to be flagged using interpretive codes, before these were synthesized to produce the final findings as presented below.

## Findings

### Work Programme theory and assumptions

Our analysis of the policy papers, ministerial statements and related documents allowed us to identify the key features of the Work Programme and its underlying assumptions that have a particular bearing on our focus of interest, namely whether and how the health-related needs of claimants will be met within this emergent provision. Overall, in common with other commentators (Lindsay and Dutton 2013; Beatty *et al.* 2013; Warren *et al.* 2011), we found that ill-health was not a prominent theme within the Work Programme policy material (see DWP 2011a). There tended to be a lack of detail in relation to health within the documents. For instance, while the policy documents stated that claimants who experience 'serious' effects from their health condition will not be expected to engage in work-related activities or work (see the Work Programme specification, DWP 2010b: 37), there was no detail on what might constitute a 'serious' effect and no health conditions were specifically defined. Furthermore, the overall message within the policy papers and ministerial discourse was that ill-health does not represent a major barrier to employment for most people and that simple interventions can support claimants with 'common health conditions' (again, not defined) into work. For instance, Freud (2011) was found to frequently cite Waddell's and Burton's (2004) evidence stating that their findings showed, 'more than 90 per cent of people with common health problems can be helped back to work by simple healthcare and workplace management measures' (Freud 2011).

There was also a tendency to locate the cause of health-related unemployment with individuals' inability to manage their condition and thereby to ignore the role a hostile labour market can play in making securing and sustaining employment difficult for those with long-term health problems. Other considerations, such as the fact that poor quality work can exacerbate some health conditions (Benach and Muntaner 2007), were also absent from the Work Programme documentation. A further key feature of the Work Programme that contrasts with its predecessor, PtW, has been its lack of prescription, for example, no health-related support provision such as CMPs. Primes were given the freedom to design and deliver provision as they saw fit in order to meet claimants' needs. This approach is referred to as black box commissioning (DWP 2011a). In relation to supporting claimants' health-related needs, DWP tender documents stated that bidders should describe their intentions to tailor support and the customer journey to meet the needs of any 'disabled customers or those with health conditions' (DWP 2010b: 38). Primes were expected to determine the type of health-related support and intervention that could help claimants with health conditions move into and sustain work, as illustrated here:

> Providers will have considerable freedom to determine what activities each customer will undertake in order to help them into, and to sustain, employment. Specialist delivery partners from the public, private and voluntary sectors are best placed to identify the best ways of getting people back to work, and will be allowed the freedom to do so without detailed prescription from central government (DWP 2010b: 6)

This excerpt also conveys a further Work Programme principle closely linked to non-prescription, namely 'personalization'. Work Programme policy documents conveyed the expectation for Primes to tailor the support provided to the needs and circumstances of individual claimants, including those with health-related barriers to employment:

> The new Work Programme will be an improvement on the current offer. It will deliver long-lasting tailored support. We are taking the first steps towards developing a package of support that includes a simplified benefits system that works alongside personalized back to work provision to support people into sustained employment (Grayling 2010)

In common with PtW, the Work Programme policy retained a core focus on the PA role. There has also been the expectation that this individual will be central to assessing individual needs and ensuring an appropriately tailored package of support and required work-related activity (upon which benefits payments are conditional) for each claimant including those with long-term ill-health. 'The role of PAs in provider organizations will be crucial in the effective delivery of the

Work Programme' (House of Commons Work and Pensions Committee 2011b: 13). Furthermore, the differential payments made available for each of the nine claimant groups has been expected to discourage Primes from focusing on those claimants who are easier to get into work and neglecting the 'harder-to-help', so-called 'creaming and parking' (Rees *et al.* 2014). Policy documents have also suggested that this payment model will prompt innovative practice, including in-work support, to meet the needs of those experiencing health-related difficulties, as the following quote indicates:

> What we will find, as the Work Programme progresses, is that providers will not only support claimants into employment but, in order to secure the larger fees, will continue to deliver support for some time after people start work. [ ... ]. I believe this will lead to providers developing new ways to support people with health conditions at work (Freud 2011)

The Work Programme policy documents also anticipated that a non-prescriptive approach would encourage Primes to draw in appropriate skills and support from other agencies and organizations in their local areas. 'This approach [the Black Box] encourages Work Programme providers to form partnerships with other organizations such as local authorities, health service providers and colleges that have an interest in helping people to move into work and to stay in work' (DWP 2011a: 9). It is important to note that, in contrast to PtW, the Work Programme policy was generated by the DWP without any formal involvement of the Department of Health and without a clearly defined role for the NHS. Therefore, any partnerships between the NHS and Primes and their sub-contractors would need to be established on a case-by-case basis.

The discussion above highlights some core assumptions of the Work Programme revealed by our analysis of the policy documents, including that:

- Primes, their sub-contractors, and particularly PAs, will have the skills and expertise to assess claimants' health-related needs and provide an appropriately tailored offer of support to each claimant.
- Primes will have the expertise to determine which health-focused interventions are effective and cost-effective at helping claimants move into and sustain work and will innovate in this area.
- Primes will be able to establish partnerships with the NHS and other agencies to secure the health-related interventions that their claimants need.

Underpinning these assumptions was an ideological position that sees large numbers of people being in receipt of sickness-related benefits as a highly undesirable situation and an avoidable drain on the public purse. Furthermore, free-market competition is viewed as the best way to establish effective solutions to this problem. The Work Programme policy documentation was found to be further suffused in a rhetoric that constructs health-related unemployment as relatively easy to address.

## Work Programme Provision: Supporting Claimants' Health-related Needs

The analysis above suggests some key areas that deserve scrutiny within the Primes' responsive bids, including:

- the extent to which the need to address claimants' health-related barriers is recognized and prioritized;
- how claimants' health-related needs will be assessed and appropriate responses identified;
- the role of PAs and their preparedness in relation to addressing health issues;
- the health condition management interventions to be made available to claimants with health conditions; and
- how functioning partnerships with NHS organizations will be established.

More generally, questions are raised in relation to the degree of variability and potential inequity in provision across contract package areas, particularly since claimants are unable to choose their Prime.

### Prominence of health

All of the 18 Primes included some reference to claimants' health-related needs, with most making reference to local health profiles at some point. However, we found varied prominence and a lack of consistent detail. Scrutiny of the Primes' minimum service levels provides a useful indication of the prominence given to claimants' health. Only five of these made explicit reference to addressing claimants' health-related needs, as shown in table 1. The lack of reference to addressing health within the majority of these summaries raises queries regarding which claimants might receive an offer of health-related support in practice, or be in a position to request such support. Since minimum service levels form part of the basis upon which the DWP monitors performance against contracts (House of Commons Work and Pensions Committee 2011a), it seems likely that most Primes will not routinely be assessed on the adequacy of their provision of health-related support.

### Assessment and claimants' Work Programme journey

Assessment of claimants' health conditions is important because it can help to identify their health-related barriers to employment. Variability in the way in which Primes proposed to use claimant assessments was evident. Assessments described included: initial, ongoing, pre-work and in-work, and some of these were specifically health-related, as shown in

135

Table 1

Explicit reference to supporting claimants' health in Primes' summarized minimum service levels (five out of 18 organizations)

| Prime reference to health | |
| --- | --- |
| A4e | 'Health support: we will assess health as a barrier to working. Those identified as needing additional assessment/support will be referred to a specialized health assessment and support to develop a health-focused back to work plan.' |
| CDG (since merged with Shaw Trust) | 'Stage Four: Pre-Employment Preparation<br>1, Customers with health problems or caring responsibilities are to be offered Work Programme support through a community hub or alternative convenient location, including home visits where required.' |
| G4S | 'Every Customer will have access to the G4S Knowledge Bank. Many Customers will require expert additional intervention to overcome barriers to finding and sustaining employment. All Customers have access to specialist Knowledge Bank services. This includes a range of support including condition management, occupational health support, childcare services, career advice, mentoring, debt advice, housing advice and vocational training.' |
| Maximus | 'Phase Three – Assessment<br>All customers undertake an assessment with a dedicated EC [Employment Coach] or Health Officer.' |
| Serco | 'Refer you to one of our specialist providers if you have particular needs, such as a health condition or physical disability, or want specific employment advice, such as how to start your own business.' |

*Note:* 13 out of 18 Primes made no explicit reference to addressing claimants' health prior to starting work in their minimum service levels (DWP 2011c: 1–14).

table 2. All of the described Work Programme journeys differed, but there were similar claimant stages and processes regardless of benefit type. A generalized Work Programme journey is presented in figure 1 to illustrate typical programme stages which ranged from three (e.g. Serco 2011) to six (e.g. Maximus 2011). The minimum frequency of claimants' appointments was defined in the Primes' minimum service levels, and was found to range from every two weeks (e.g. Seetec 2011) to once a month (e.g. A4e 2011). Health-related intervention might be offered at any stage in these journeys, as shown by the asterisks in figure 1, and there was no consistency across Primes in this regard. In keeping with the principle of personalization, several bids emphasized

Table 2

Primes' bid statements (2011) in relation to claimant assessment process

| Prime | Initial assessment process | Mentioned health barriers | Initial assessment carried out by | Initial health assessments available through filtering process* | Health assessment carried out by |
|---|---|---|---|---|---|
| A4E | Initial call from customer support centre to discuss needs. Dialogue-driven assessment | ✓ | PA | Specialist health assessments which aim to identify capacity to work | Healthcare professionals from advanced personnel management |
| Avanta | Face-to-face dialogue driven. Use of online and paper-based assessment tools and diagnostics | X | PA | X | X |
| BEST (now Interserve) | A range of diagnostic tests to inform the initial assessment. Use of Rickter Scale | ✓ | Customer service consultant then PA | Occupational health assessments pre-work | A physiotherapist and nurse |
| CDG (since merged with Shaw Trust) | Initial phone triage assessment. Self-assessment: a brief questionnaire. Work-focused assessment: via interview | X | An adviser Claimant PA | X | X |
| ESG Holdings Limited | Diagnostic assessment tool. Two-part assessment: an online psychometric questionnaire and structured interview | ✓ | Trained assessor PA | X | X |
| EOS (formerly FourstaR Employment and Skills Ltd) | Market-tested diagnostic. The Work Star and own diagnostics | X | PA | In-depth assessment of work capability | In-house work health expert role |

(continued)

Table 2

(*Continued*)

| Prime | Initial assessment process | Mentioned health barriers | Initial assessment carried out by | Initial health assessments available through filtering process* | Health assessment carried out by |
|---|---|---|---|---|---|
| G4S | Diagnostics | ✓ | PA | Specific needs assessment tools such as mental health first aid and hidden disabilities diagnostics | Subcontractor advisers; mind and dyslexia action |
| Ingeus UK Limited | Online self-diagnosis tool Diagnostics | X | Claimant with guidance from PA | Where relevant to assess workplace capabilities | In-house healthcare professionals (health advisers – physical and mental health) |
| JHP | Bespoke screening tool and further in-depth assessment | ✓ | Customer Service Administrator then PA | X | X |
| Maximus | Initial screening with self-assessment online where possible 1:1 with an employment consultant using web tool, or with a health consultant | X | Claimant PA | Claimants with '*serious health issues*' limiting their ability to get a job (:14) | Mobile health consultant led via the in-house health team |

| | | | | Enhanced assessments indicated such as mental health assessments | Specialist partner organizations |
|---|---|---|---|---|---|
| NCG | Personalized, psychological and motivational intervention over 2 days. Followed by an employability assessment | ✓ | PA | X | X |
| Pertemps People Development Group | Employability diagnostic and further diagnostic assessment | X | PA | X | X |
| Prospects | Initial assessment by phone then a face-to-face assessment | ✓ | PA | X | X |
| Reed | Diagnostics tool and progression model | X | PA | X | X |
| Rehab JobFit | Specialist assessments conducted in different situations including groups | ✓ | PA | X | X |
| Seetec | Face-to-face or telephone/online. Online self-assessment questionnaires, then solution-focused interviewing | ✓ | PA | X | X |
| Serco | In-depth assessment process | ✓ | PA | X | X |
| Working Links | Diagnostic assessment | ✓ | PA | X | X |

*Notes:* ✓ = identified in bid document; X = not identified in bid document; * = excludes statements relating to specialist assessments which could potentially include health.

Figure 1

Generalized work programme journey

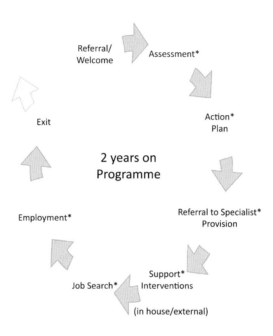

that the frequency of contact and speed of movement through the claimant journey would depend upon individual need and progress.

## Personal advisers

All of the Primes outlined a PA role which was typically described as central to supporting claimants' progress into, and sustainment in, work. The extent to which a PA was indicated to stay with a claimant across the whole journey varied. Fourteen Primes showed a preference for continuity, aiming to ensure that claimants would have a 'dedicated' PA, and in some cases terming this 'case management' (e.g. CDG 2011). In contrast, a split model, which was adopted by Serco, intentionally aims to ensure that claimants change PAs during their Work Programme journey, arguing that this 'challenges comfort zones' and provides 'extra impetus' (Serco 2011: 17).

A range of PA role titles were identified and although there were similarities across the bid documents, this role was not found to be standardized. Five out of 18 Primes included some mention of specialist PAs with health-related roles. However, there was a good deal of variation in the type of specialist skills mentioned, for instance 'mental health awareness' versus 'cognitive behavioural therapy'. A variety of other specialist roles were also identified in the documents, but it was difficult to clarify the exact nature of their expertise and whether or not they would have a heath focus. Some Primes such as EOS and Working Links indicated that they would provide health-related training to all PAs, others to only some. However, the extent to which such training will prepare and equip PAs to support claimants' health-related barriers is difficult to assess.

## Health-focused interventions

*Healthcare professional roles.*   Only four out of the 18 Primes documented in-house healthcare professional roles as part of their delivery model (A4e 2011; EOS 2011; Ingeus UK Limited 2011; Maximus 2011). Despite different titles – health adviser, health consultant, occupational health coach and work health expert – further examination of these roles suggested that they all are intended to have a similar combined health and work focus. Three of these roles also have a requirement to support PAs: A4e, Ingeus UK Limited and Maximus. Clarifying whether Primes' health-related interventions would be delivered by healthcare professionals, or someone else, was not always possible. For example, Prospects (2011) stated that it will provide 'well being groups' but it was not clear who would deliver these (Prospects 2011: 11). Investigations of sub-contractor/partner websites helped in some cases to identify the healthcare professional roles that might be involved as shown in table 2.

*Condition management.*   All of the Primes referred to some kind of health-management intervention, but there was variability across Primes in terms of which claimants would be eligible for receipt of these interventions. It was unclear how such eligibility criteria would be defined or operationalized in practice, but bids suggest some kind of prioritization or rationing of the interventions. Fifteen out of the 18 bids used the term 'condition management' to refer to health-related interventional support, but there appeared to be significant variation in terms of the content of the interventions on offer. Interventional approaches included: cognitive behavioural therapy, solution-focused therapy, counselling and motivational interviewing techniques. What might be perceived as more clinical interventions ('hands on') such as physiotherapy were also mentioned in a minority of the bids. Health-management interventions included: advice and guidance (such as pain management techniques), promotion of healthy lifestyles and encouragement of activities such as walking and healthy diets (e.g. Ingeus UK Limited 2011). More complementary health-related interventions such as yoga and Tai Chi were also proposed by one Prime (EOS 2011). Importantly, some bids included mention of interventions involving employers to explore workplace adjustments and proposed provision of ongoing condition management support post-employment (e.g. A4e 2011). These varied interventions were planned to be carried out through group work and/or one to one, via face-to-face in a range of venues and locations, or via telephone support services.

141

Arrangements for provision of these health-management interventions varied amongst Primes, with some proposing to make use of existing statutory health-related provision for example A4e (2011), while others intended to provide them in-house. All of the 18 Primes proposed the use of a range of specialist providers, and many of these are indicated to be used in an ad hoc fashion as and when claimants' needs arise.

*NHS partnerships.* The DWP encouraged Primes to demonstrate in their bids an awareness of local provision to avoid duplicating services and develop effective partnerships (DWP 2010a), including with local health services. Table 3 provides an overview of the Primes' statements about their proposed NHS partnerships and engagement. As shown, half of the Primes indicated they had an established connection with the NHS, which had been developed through an existing programme or their supply chain. For example, Serco highlighted that one of its sub-contractors (Yes2 Ventures) has links with GPs, 'South Yorkshire Condition Management (Yes2Ventures) works with 104 GP practices across Sheffield' (Serco 2011: 20). However, table 3 also shows that it was more common for Primes to have stated an intention to consult with NHS stakeholders when designing their programme, rather than to have already developed specific plans for co-location or commissioning of services at the bidding stage.

## Discussion

The review sought to generate insight into the Work Programme national policy and how it is being operationalized by Primes via an interpretive documentary review. It is important to recognize that any documentary review can only provide a partial picture of public policy and its translation into practice. It was evident that many details were lacking within the Primes' bid documents and therefore that elements of health-related provision may have been overlooked or misunderstood in this review. On the other hand, recent research has revealed that some elements mentioned in the bids have not been forthcoming in practice (Lane *et al.* 2013). Notwithstanding these limitations, the review does provide valuable information about what the DWP considered to be acceptable in terms of proposed health-related support. It also serves to identify a number of potential risks and opportunities that deserve attention as the programme is rolled out and evaluative research is undertaken.

It is important to highlight first a number of general issues that relate to the overall design of the Work Programme and the implications for the health-related support that is offered to claimants across the country. Overall, the bid documents acknowledged that claimants' health-related issues can become barriers to employment, suggesting that this dimension was considered within their broad delivery model. However, the allocation of DWP contracts to a large number of Primes with

Table 3

Summary of Primes' bid statements (2011) in relation to proposed National Health Service partnerships and engagement strategies

| Prime | Existing relationship | Initial talks held | Continue engagement | Plans to: Co-locate services | Align services | Co-commission | Other statements |
|---|---|---|---|---|---|---|---|
| A4e | ✓ | ✓ | ✓ | ✓ | ✓ | | |
| Avanta | | ✓ | | ✓ | | | |
| BEST | ✓ | | ✓ | | | | |
| CDG | ✓ | ✓ | ✓ | | | | |
| EOS | | ✓ | ✓ | | | | |
| ESG Holdings Limited | | ✓ | ✓ | | | | |
| G4S | | | ✓ | | | | |
| Ingeus | | | | ✓ | ✓ | ✓ | |
| JHP | | | ✓ | | | | |
| Maximus | ✓ | | ✓ | | | | ✓1 |
| NCG | | | ✓ | | | | ✓2 |
| Pertemps People Development Group | ✓ | | ✓ | | | | |
| Prospects | ✓ | | ✓ | | | | |
| Reed | ✓ | ✓ | | | ✓ | | |
| Rehab JobFit | ✓ | ✓ | ✓ | | | | ✓3 |
| Seetec | ✓ | | ✓ | | | | |
| Serco | ✓ | | | | ✓ | | |
| Working Links | | | | | | | ✓4 |

*Notes:* ✓ = relates to section 7.1 of the bid document; some Primes state more general plans to have ongoing engagement with known stakeholders which may include the NHS: ✓1 = to join with NHS services; ✓2 = to provide in-house space for NHS trainers to deliver their services; ✓3 = nothing identified that was specific; ✓4 = will work with health/specialist provider organizations.

minimal prescription has resulted in very varied delivery models and content across contract package areas. Further, since some Primes also operate as sub-contractors for other Primes in different contract package areas, different service offers to claimants are provided even by the same provider organization. The result is a highly variable offer and the potential for significant inequity within the system. Individuals facing similar health-related obstacles to employment can expect to receive very different levels and types of support depending on which Primes' programme they are assigned to join. Further, the lack of prescription around minimum service levels means that very few of the Primes will be explicitly performance managed against health-related support. The extent to which this commissioning model will encourage innovation or more effective support models for claimants with health-related needs remains to be seen.

Primes appear to have responded to the DWP's call to establish partnership arrangements and thereby draw on local resources and expertise to meet claimant needs. However, the resultant sub-contracting arrangements appear to be highly complex and it was not possible to clarify the exact details regarding health-management intervention delivery from the bid documents. This lack of clarity in successful bids suggests that there was limited scrutiny of the adequacy and feasibility of proposed arrangements on the part of DWP commissioners. Emerging evidence supports concerns that sub-contracting arrangements are highly variable and inconsistent with expected patterns in practice (see Lane *et al.* 2013; Newton *et al.* 2012; Kerr 2013). This suggests the need for further investigation into the health-related support provision that is materializing on the ground.

In relation to more specific elements of the delivery models, a number of issues are worth highlighting. In common with earlier work (Coleman and Parry 2011), our analysis suggests significant variation in the form and use of claimant assessment procedures across Primes. This raises questions about the consistency with which individual health-related barriers will be recognized and responded to. In particular, many of the Primes intended to 'spot purchase' specialist health management input from sub-contractors for claimants deemed in need of such support. Typically, access to such provision was often at the discretion of PAs and highly dependent on the organizations' assessment processes, raising the potential for claimants' health-related needs to be inadequately identified, or missed. Given that some health conditions can be hidden, PAs' expertise in assessing claimants' health-related barriers to employment is likely to be essential.

PAs were central to the Work Programme delivery across all Primes, and there was an expectation that they would be able to support claimants with health conditions. However, there were inconsistencies in whether, and how, Primes would ensure their PAs were adequately skilled and trained to respond to claimants' health-related needs. This is of concern because only a minority of Primes made explicit reference to having in-house healthcare professionals to support PAs.

Co-location of PAs and healthcare professionals has been shown to provide a number of advantages, enabling some PAs to become more knowledgeable about healthcare professionals' practice (Lindsay and Dutton 2012) and claimants' health-related needs (Barnes and Hudson 2006). Therefore, questions are raised about how PAs are practicing if they have not received adequate health training, and no healthcare professional support is available.

In fact, only four of the 18 Primes actually proposed an in-house healthcare professional role and it is not yet known how many of these in-house roles are available in practice. There were unanswered questions about how some of the health-related provision, (in-house and external led) would be provided. The proposed limited involvement of healthcare professionals in the delivery models suggests that some Primes may opt to address claimants' health-related needs with non-clinical staff, a pattern that was also evident within some of the PtW CMPs (Nice and Davidson 2010). Although this approach was not necessarily considered to be ineffective, supervisory structures are important (Nice and Davidson 2010). It remains unclear whether these will be established within the Work Programme. This raises a set of questions relating to both risk to claimants and value for money, as cheaper models may not be as cost-effective if outcomes are poor.

There were also variations in whether Primes stated they had worked, or intended to work in partnership with the NHS. Vague statements suggested underdeveloped relationships in some contract package areas. For instance, while some bids were clear about their intentions to support claimants to access NHS provision, there was minimal awareness that demand for these services might exceed supply. Additionally, it was uncommon for Primes to state that they would consider paying for additional services that might be needed. As there are a large number of Work Programme providers operating within each geographical area (i.e. Primes and sub-contractors), navigation is likely to be time consuming. Therefore, exploration of how care for claimants can be integrated at a system level, including referral pathways and payment mechanisms is clearly needed.

The bid review identified that all Primes intended to offer health-management interventions to at least some of their claimants, often via subcontracting arrangements. While it is not possible to comment on the effectiveness of the proposed interventions, the wide variety of descriptors raises questions regarding the quality, adequacy and equity of services provided to different claimants. Uncertainty also exists regarding eligibility criteria since several Primes employed additional eligibility descriptors such as 'severe' or 'serious' and these may be poorly defined and variably understood in practice. Whether support will be rationed for those deemed to be in most need or closer to starting work deserves future investigation. On the other hand, some Primes stated their intention to make health-related support available for all claimants and yet appear to have made minimal provision, raising concerns about demand-supply mismatch.

On a more positive note, there appears to be some promising innovation, for example the offer of bespoke CMPs by one Prime (EOS 2011). This suggests that claimants will receive support for a range of health conditions rather than prioritizing interventions for musculoskeletal, cardiorespiratory and mild to moderate mental health, as was the earlier pattern in PtW. There also appeared to be further innovation with the inclusion of telephone support interventions which have been found to be both effective and cost-effective (Burton *et al.* 2013). Telephone interventions may also reduce claimants' anxieties and concerns about sharing their problems in a group setting and the problems associated with having to travel to venues which were highlighted as potential barriers in the PtW CMP (Nice and Davidson 2010). Ongoing and longer-term support was another gap in the PtW CMP and this was addressed in some bids through proposed in-work support interventions. Given the competitive nature of the Work Programme contracts, there may be a lack of willingness to share best practice amongst Primes, which may limit service developments. However, there is scope for Primes to find out what interventions are working well in those areas where they also operate as subcontractors. Therefore variations in Primes' offers may lessen over time.

## Conclusion

Through the adoption of the black box approach, Primes have been given considerable leeway in designing their delivery. The resultant high variability in health-related support means that claimants with similar health conditions are likely to experience very different levels of service. When reconsidering the three assumptions identified above, it appears likely that some Primes and PAs may not be equipped to assess and respond to claimants' health-related needs. This is important because the PA role was central to much of the proposed Work Programme delivery, yet concerns have been raised regarding their preparedness and training in assessing and addressing claimants' health-related needs. Given there are known pressures in terms of some PAs having high caseload numbers and struggles in the financing of programmes, there is an increasing need to ensure that Work Programme assessment processes are effective (Newton *et al.* 2012; House of Commons Work and Pensions Committee 2013). Integration with appropriate healthcare professionals and provision is therefore likely to be essential, but is currently under-developed.

Some Primes have shown promise of designing innovative interventions, but it is not known if these will be effective and/or cost-effective. Given there were variations in whether Primes stated they had worked, or intended to work in partnership, with the NHS, claimants' access to health-related provision may be limited. Thus, the review's findings question whether the Work Programme policy is sufficiently health-focused and whether the black box commissioning approach can stimulate innovation in effective health-related approaches.

Importantly, while policy rhetoric has implied that claimants' health problems are easy to address, the latest research evaluations and evidence reveal poor outcomes for many claimants who have health-related needs (House of Commons Work and Pensions Committee 2013; Newton *et al.* 2012; Kerr 2013). Thus, policy needs to ensure that claimants' health-related barriers are adequately addressed. Research to explore whether and how Primes are operating on the ground to address claimants' health-related needs in practice is now a priority.

## Acknowledgements

This study was funded by the National Institute for Health Research, Collaboration for Leadership in Applied Health Research and Care for South Yorkshire (NIHR CLAHRC SY), which acknowledges funding from the NIHR. The views and opinions expressed are those of the authors, and not necessarily those of the NHS, the NIHR or the Department of Health. CLAHRC SY would also like to acknowledge the participation and resources of our partner organizations. Further details can be found at the CLAHRC SY website, http://www.clahrc-sy.nihr.ac.uk.

## References

A4e (2011), *Employment related support services framework agreement mini competitions for the provision of the Work Programme invitation to tender form*, CPA 06, http:// www.contractsfinder.businesslink.gov.uk (accessed 26 June 2012).

Avanta Enterprise Ltd (Avanta) (2011), *Employment related support services framework agreement mini competitions for the provision of the Work Programme invitation to tender form*, CPA 05, http://www.contractsfinder.businesslink.gov.uk (accessed 26 June 2012).

Barnes, H. and Hudson, M. (2006), *Pathways to Work – Extension to some Existing Customers Early Findings from Qualitative Research*, Department for Work and Pensions Research Report 323, Leeds: Corporate Document Services.

Beatty, C. and Fothergill, S. (2011), *Incapacity benefits in the UK: An issue of health or jobs?* Paper given at Social Policy Association Annual Conference, Lincoln, UK, 4–6 July.

Beatty, C., Duncan, K., Fothergill, S. and McLean, S. (2013), *The Role of Health Interventions in Reducing Incapacity Claimant Numbers*, Sheffield: Sheffield Hallam University, http://www.shu.ac.uk/research/cresr/sites/shu.ac.uk/files/health-interventions-incapacity-claimant.pdf (accessed 11 November 2013).

Benach, J. and Muntaner, C. (2007), Precarious employment and health: developing a research agenda, *Journal of Epidemiology and Community Health*, 61, 4: 276–7.

Black, C. and Frost, D. (2011), *Health at Work – An Independent Review of Sickness Absence*, Cm 8205, London: The Stationery Office.

Burton, K., Kendall, N., McCluskey, S. and Dibben, P. (2013), *Telephonic Support to Facilitate Return to Work: What Works, How, and When?* Research Report 853, Sheffield: Department for Work and Pensions.

Business Employment Services Ltd (BEST) (2011), *Employment related support services framework agreement mini competitions for the provision of the Work*

*Programme invitation to tender form*, CPA 16, http://www.contractsfinder .businesslink.gov.uk (accessed 26 June 2012).

Careers Development Group (CDG) (2011), *Employment related support services framework agreement mini competitions for the provision of the Work Programme invitation to tender form*, CPA 04, http://www.contractsfinder.businesslink.gov.uk (accessed 26 June 2012).

Coleman, N. and Parry, F. (2011), *Opening up Work for All. The Role of Assessment in the Work Programme*, London: Centre for Economic and Social Inclusion.

Department for Work and Pensions (DWP) (2002), *Pathways to Work: Helping People into Employment*, Cm 5690, London: Stationery Office.

Department for Work and Pensions (DWP) (2010a), *Building Bridges to Work: New Approaches to Tackling Long-term Worklessness*, Cm 7817, London: The Stationery Office.

Department for Work and Pensions (DWP) (2010b), *The Work Programme Invitation to Tender Specification and Supporting Information*, Sheffield: DWP.

Department for Work and Pensions (DWP) (2010c), *Employment Related Support Services Framework Agreement Mini Competitions for the Provision of the Work Programme Instructions for Bidders*, Sheffield: DWP.

Department for Work and Pensions (DWP) (2011a), *The Work Programme*, https://www.gov.uk/government/uploads/system/uploads/attachment_da ta/file/49884/the-work-programme.pdf (accessed 10 September 2011).

Department for Work and Pensions (DWP) (2011b), In: House of Commons Work and Pensions Committee (2011), *Work Programme: Providers and Contracting Arrangements*, HC 718 (2010–12), London: The Stationery Office.

Department for Work and Pensions (DWP) (2011c), *Minimum Service Delivery*, http://webarchive.nationalarchives.gov.uk/+/http://dwp.gov.uk/docs/ provider-minimum-service-delivery.pdf (accessed 20 November 2013).

Dickens, S., Mowlam, A. and Woodfield, K. (2004), *Incapacity Benefit Reforms – The PA Role & Practices*, DWP Research Report 212, Leeds: Corporate Document Services.

EOS (2011), *Employment related support services framework agreement mini competitions for the provision of the Work Programme invitation to tender form*, CPA 14, http://www.contractsfinder.businesslink.gov.uk (accessed 26 June 2012) (EOS: formerly FourstaR Employment and Skills Ltd).

ESG Holdings Limited (2011), *Employment related support services framework agreement mini competitions for the provision of the Work Programme invitation to tender form*, CPA 15, http://www.contractsfinder.businesslink.gov.uk (accessed 26 June 2012).

Freud, D. (2011), *Health and Wellbeing*, Speech given at the Govnet Health and Well-being Conference, London, UK, 6 October.

Grayling, C. (2010), Speech given at the Welfare to Work Event, Centre for Economic and Social Inclusion, London, UK, 1 July.

G4S (2011), *Employment related support services framework agreement mini competitions for the provision of the Work Programme invitation to tender form*, CPA 10, http:// www.contractsfinder.businesslink.gov.uk (accessed 26 June 2012).

House of Commons Work and Pensions Committee (2011a), *Work Programme: Providers and Contracting Arrangements*, HC 718 (2010–12), London: The Stationery Office.

House of Commons Work and Pensions Committee (2011b), *Work Programme: Providers and Contracting Arrangements: Government Response to the Committee's Fourth Report of Session 2010–12*, HC 1438 (2010–12), London: The Stationery Office.

House of Commons Work and Pensions Committee (2013), *Can the Work Programme Work for all User Groups?* HC 162 (2013–14), London: The Stationery Office.

Ingeus UK Limited (2011), *Employment related support services framework agreement mini competitions for the provision of the Work Programme invitation to tender form*, CPA 02, http://www.contractsfinder.businesslink.gov.uk (accessed 26 June 2012).

JHP Group Ltd (JHP) (2011), *Employment related support services framework agreement mini competitions for the provision of the Work Programme invitation to tender form*, CPA 12, http://www.contractsfinder.businesslink.gov.uk (accessed 26 June 2012).

Jobcentre Plus (2006), *Condition Management Programmes: What Are They, What is the Evidence Base, What do they Currently Look Like?* http://www.jobcentreplus.gov.uk/JCP/stellent/groups/jcp/documents/websitecontent/dev012591.doc (accessed 8 October 2007).

Kellett, S., Bickerstaffe, D., Purdie, F., Dyke, A., Filer, S., Lomax, V. and Tomlinson, H. (2011), The clinical and occupational effectiveness of condition management for Incapacity Benefit recipients, *British Journal of Clinical Psychology*, 50, 2: 164–77.

Kemp, P. A. and Davidson, J. (2010), Employability trajectories among new claimants of incapacity benefit, *Policy Studies*, 3, 2: 203–21.

Kerr, S. (2013), *Fair Chance to Work 2 Experiences from the First Phase of the Work Programme Delivery in London*, London: London Voluntary Service Council.

Lane, P., Foster, R., Gardiner, L., Lanceley, L. and Purvis, A. (2013), *Work Programme Evaluation: Procurement, Supply Chains and Implementation of the Commissioning Model*, Department for Work and Pensions Research Report No 832, London: Department for Work and Pensions.

Lindsay, C. and Dutton, M. (2010), Employability through health? Partnership-based governance and the delivery of Pathways to Work condition management services, *Policy Studies*, 31, 2: 245–64.

Lindsay, C. and Dutton, M. (2012), Promoting healthy routes back to work? Boundary spanning health professionals and employability programmes in Great Britain, *Social Policy & Administration*, 46, 5: 509–25.

Lindsay, C. and Dutton, M. (2013), Promoting healthy pathways to employability: lessons for the UK's welfare-to-work agenda, *Policy and Politics*, 4, 2: 183–200.

Maximus Employment UK Limited (Maximus) (2011), *Employment related support services framework agreement mini competitions for the provision of the Work Programme invitation to tender form*, CPA 09, http://www.contractsfinder.businesslink.gov.uk (accessed 26 June 2012).

Morestin, F., Gauvin, P., Hogue, M. and Benoit, F. (2010), *Method for Synthesizing Knowledge about Public Policies, Montreal:* National Collaborating Centre for Healthy Public Policy.

National Audit Office (2012), *The Introduction of the Work Programme*, HC 1701 (2010–12), London: The Stationery Office.

Newcastle College Group (NCG) (2011), *Employment related support services framework agreement mini competitions for the provision of the Work Programme invitation to tender form*, CPA 18, http://www.contractsfinder.businesslink.gov.uk (accessed 26 June 2012).

Newton, B., Meager, N., Bertram, C., Corden, A., George, A., Lalani, M., Metcalf, H., Rolfe, H., Sainsbury, R. and Weston, K. (2012), *Work Programme Evaluation: Findings from the First Phase of Qualitative Research on Programme Delivery*,

Department for Work and Pensions Research Report No 821, London: Department for Work and Pensions.

Nice, K. and Davidson, J. (2010), *Provider Led Pathways: Experiences and Views of Condition Management Programme*, Department for Work and Pensions Research Report No 644, Leeds: Corporate Document Services.

Pertemps People Development Group (2011), *Employment related support services framework agreement mini competitions for the provision of the Work Programme invitation to tender form*, CPA 14, http://www.contractsfinder.businesslink.gov.uk (accessed 26 June 2012).

Prior, L. (2008), Repositioning documents in social research, *Sociology*, 42, 5: 821–36.

Prospects (2011), *Employment related support services framework agreement mini competitions for the provision of the Work Programme invitation to tender form*, CPA 11, http:// www.contractsfinder.businesslink.gov.uk (accessed 26 June 2012).

Randall, E. (2011), *The DWP Funded and NHS Delivered Condition Management Programme: Lessons Learned*, Sheffield: Department for Work and Pensions.

Reed (2011), *Employment related support services framework agreement mini competitions for the provision of the Work Programme invitation to tender form*, CPA 03, http:// www.contractsfinder.businesslink.gov.uk (accessed 26 June 2012).

Rees, J., Whitworth, A. and Carter, E. (2014), Support for all in the UK work programme? Differential payments, same old problem, *Social Policy & Administration*, 48, 2: 221–39.

Rehab JobFit LLP (Rehab JobFit) (2011), *Employment related support services framework agreement mini competitions for the provision of the Work Programme invitation to tender form*, CPA 13, http://www.contractsfinder.businesslink.gov.uk (accessed 26 June 2012).

Scott, J. (1990), *A Matter of Record*, Cambridge: Polity Press.

Seetec (2011), *Employment related support services framework agreement mini competitions for the provision of the Work Programme invitation to tender form*, CPA 07, http:// www.contractsfinder.businesslink.gov.uk (accessed 26 June 2012).

Serco (2011), *Employment related support services framework agreement mini competitions for the provision of the Work Programme invitation to tender form*, CPA 17, http:// www.contractsfinder.businesslink.gov.uk (accessed 26 June 2012).

Shaw, S., Elston, J. and Abbott, S. (2004), Comparative analysis of health policy implementation: the use of documentary analysis, *Policy Studies*, 25, 4: 259–66.

Stafford, B. (2012), Supporting moves into work: New Deal for Disabled People findings, *Scandinavian Journal of Disability Research*, 14, 2: 165–76.

Waddell, G. and Burton, K. (2004), *Concepts of Rehabilitation for the Management of Common Health Problems*, London: The Stationery Office.

Warren, J., Garthwaite, K. and Bambra, C. (2011), *A Health Problem? Health and Employability in the UK Labour Market*, Paper given at the Health, Employability and Challenges for Welfare Reform Symposium at the Social Policy Association Conference, Lincoln, UK, 4–6 July.

Working Links (2011), *Employment related support services framework agreement mini competitions for the provision of the Work Programme invitation to tender form*, CPA 13, http://www.contractsfinder.businesslink.gov.uk (accessed 26 June 2012).

# 8

# *Supporting the UK's Workless – An International Comparative Perspective*

## Mike Danson[*], Ailsa McKay and Willie Sullivan

## Introduction

Poverty and ill health remain a scourge in the lives of many in modern, capitalist societies, despite wealth and income at the national and global level rising over the decades. The persistence of such deprivations are not inevitable but rather are down to the choices made by governments and societies:

> 'Why do we have less poverty than the United States, but much more than Norway, Sweden and Denmark?' (Brady, 2009, 5). The reasons lie very much more in the distribution systems of the respective countries than in the personal behaviour of people in poverty. 'Why some affluent Western democracies maintain substantial poverty and others are more egalitarian and accomplish low levels of poverty' is mainly due to 'the generosity of the welfare state (Brady, 2009, 166)' (Sinfield 2011: 5)

Within and between nations, spatial inequalities in relation to health, labour markets and employment shape the barriers faced by those trapped on unemployment and disability benefits, and thus create challenges for public policy. The popular discourse in the UK has become dominated by the notion that levels of social security and welfare payments are determined by what we can afford as a society, and that they have a particular and critical significance also on the supply-side of the labour market in terms of incentives and rewards (Mooney 2014). Notions of universalism have been questioned as part of this agenda and the Labour Party in Scotland, for instance, has

*New Perspectives on Health, Disability, Welfare and the Labour Market*, First Edition.
Edited by Colin Lindsay, Bent Greve, Ignazio Cabras, Nick Ellison and Stephen Kellett.
© 2015 John Wiley & Sons, Ltd. Published 2015 by John Wiley & Sons, Ltd.

appeared to forsake its previous support for delivering certain benefits to all (Lamont 2012) in contrast with the Scottish Government's approach (Salmond 2013); research with the Poverty Programme at Oxfam (Trebeck 2013; Danson and Trebeck 2013) and the Jimmy Reid Foundation (Danson *et al.* 2012) has reaffirmed the arguments for universalism in defence of this approach to social security.

By contrast, near neighbours to the UK, with similar cultures and politics and levels of economic development, have quite different systems of support for those unable to work or otherwise not in employment (Bennett 2014); and most of these countries have enjoyed better economic records over recent decades.

To provide context for such analyses and policy discussions, the second section of this article first presents evidence on levels of poverty, welfare support and inequality across Europe. It compares and contrasts especially the position and support for those out of or at the margins of the labour market under different welfare states to reveal the significant differences between the UK on the one hand and the Nordic and Benelux countries on the other hand. The third section proposes that the implications of inequalities and exclusion are of relevance to wider considerations of economic and industrial performance. In particular, this forms the basis for gathering insights from theories and practices of endogenous growth, universalism and inclusion. This allows the article to demonstrate that lessons are to be learnt from the better economic and social performances of the more inclusive and coherent nations of northern Europe. In particular, the fourth section argues that the very high levels of poverty and inequality inherent in the neo-liberal policies of the UK cannot generate the conditions for simultaneously reducing public sector deficits and stimulating demand so that worklessness and exclusion inevitably will continue. An alternative approach to social security is discussed in the fifth section. The article concludes that an alternative social democratic paradigm is required based on solidarity, equity and fiscal responsibility to address this self-defeating feedback.

## Comparative Analyses

The populism of the welfare reform agenda partly depends for its legitimacy on the claim that the UK devotes a high proportion of national income and public expenditure on social security payments. The propaganda around this is explored elsewhere in this Special Issue. However, it is revealing to compare expenditures on 'social protection' per inhabitant across the EU (figure 1). Far from the UK appearing to be profligate, both before the financial crisis really had made its effects known in 2008 and in 2010–11 (table 1), it sits in the middle of the ranking with only the poorer member states spending less on welfare than the UK and all other parts of the EU spending more (European Commission 2013). The UK spends about the EU28 average on its citizens as a proportion of its national income, with other parts of the European

Figure 1

Expenditure on social protection, 2010–11 (% of gross domestic product)

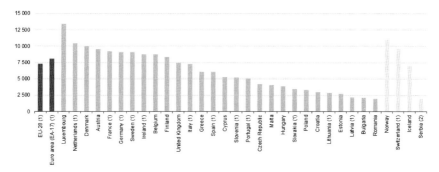

*Source:* Eurostat (online data code: tps00100), http://epp.eurostat.ec.europa.eu/statistics_explained/index.php/Social_protection_statistics (accessed 11 April 2014). *Notes:* 1 = provisional; 2 = 2010.

Economic Area also more generous (figure 1). This confirms both the different political economy playing out in this country compared with the rest of the continent and the need to interpret national statistics in wider contexts.

When the levels of income replacement for those out of work are examined, it is clear that those losing their job in the UK fare far worse relative to those in similar problems in the Nordic countries. Table 2 presents the incomes to be expected for different family types at different levels of pre-redundancy wages as a proportion of these wages. For almost all household types, the income that a family can expect after someone has lost their job in the UK is lower than their counterparts across northern Europe. Only Ireland, with a similar welfare system the UK, approaches the UK in the compensation offered. These results hold regardless of whether there are other adults in the home, children and whether the earnings before unemployment were below, at or above the national average wage. Our much earlier work on the reservation wage of the unemployed (Hunter *et al.* 1988) confirmed others' findings that British workers do not price themselves out of jobs; as the quote from Sinfield (2011) above confirms, the social security approach in the UK is punitive on spurious grounds (Bennett 2014). And, as with the statistics on the costs per head of social protection discussed above, the UK stands well down the league table for replacement rates for the unemployed when considered globally (table 3).

This is a contributory factor in the high degree of inequality in the UK (figure 2) with the country having one of the highest 'gaps' between rich and poor. This is a significant factor in the health of both society and the economy (Goulden 2012; Stiglitz 2012; Trebeck 2013). While

153

Table 1

Expenditure on social protection, 2001–11 (% of gross domestic product)

| | 2001 | 2002 | 2003 | 2004 | 2005 | 2006 | 2007 | 2008 | 2009 | 2010 | 2011 |
|---|---|---|---|---|---|---|---|---|---|---|---|
| EU_28 | : | : | : | : | : | : | : | 26.8 | 29.7 | 29.4 | 29.1 |
| EU_27 | : | : | : | : | 27.0 | 26.6 | 26.1 | 26.8 | 29.6 | 29.3 | 29.0 |
| Euro area (EA-17) | 26.8 | 27.4 | 27.7 | 27.6 | 27.7 | 27.3 | 26.9 | 27.6 | 30.4 | 30.4 | 30.0 |
| Belgium | 26.3 | 26.7 | 27.4 | 27.4 | 27.3 | 27.0 | 26.9 | 28.3 | 30.6 | 30.1 | 30.4 |
| Bulgaria | : | : | : | : | 15.1 | 14.2 | 14.1 | 15.5 | 17.2 | 18.1 | 17.7 |
| Czech Republic | 18.7 | 19.4 | 19.4 | 18.6 | 18.4 | 18.0 | 18.0 | 18.0 | 20.3 | 20.2 | 20.4 |
| Denmark | 29.2 | 29.7 | 30.9 | 30.7 | 30.2 | 29.2 | 30.7 | 30.7 | 34.7 | 34.3 | 34.3 |
| Germany | 29.7 | 30.4 | 30.8 | 30.1 | 30.1 | 29.0 | 27.8 | 28.0 | 31.5 | 30.6 | 29.4 |
| Estonia | 13.0 | 12.7 | 12.5 | 13.0 | 12.6 | 12.1 | 12.1 | 14.9 | 19.0 | 18.0 | 16.1 |
| Ireland | 14.3 | 16.7 | 17.2 | 17.4 | 17.5 | 17.8 | 18.3 | 21.5 | 26.5 | 28.5 | 29.6 |
| Greece | 24.3 | 24.0 | 23.5 | 23.6 | 24.9 | 24.8 | 24.8 | 26.2 | 28.0 | 29.1 | 30.2 |
| Spain | 19.7 | 20.0 | 20.3 | 20.3 | 20.6 | 20.5 | 20.8 | 22.2 | 25.4 | 25.8 | 26.1 |
| France (1) | 29.6 | 30.5 | 31.0 | 31.4 | 31.5 | 31.2 | 30.9 | 31.3 | 33.6 | 33.8 | 33.6 |
| Croatia | : | : | : | : | : | : | : | 18.7 | 20.8 | 21.0 | 20.6 |
| Italy | 24.8 | 25.2 | 25.7 | 25.9 | 26.3 | 26.6 | 26.6 | 27.7 | 29.9 | 29.9 | 29.7 |
| Cyprus | 14.9 | 16.3 | 18.4 | 18.1 | 18.4 | 18.5 | 18.2 | 19.5 | 21.1 | 22.1 | 22.8 |
| Latvia | 14.7 | 14.3 | 14.0 | 13.2 | 12.8 | 12.7 | 11.3 | 12.7 | 16.9 | 17.8 | 15.1 |
| Lithuania | 14.7 | 14.0 | 13.5 | 13.4 | 13.2 | 13.3 | 14.4 | 16.1 | 21.2 | 19.1 | 17.0 |
| Luxembourg | 20.9 | 21.6 | 22.1 | 22.3 | 21.7 | 20.4 | 19.3 | 21.4 | 24.3 | 23.1 | 22.5 |
| Hungary | 19.5 | 20.4 | 21.3 | 20.8 | 21.9 | 22.5 | 22.7 | 22.9 | 24.3 | 23.1 | 23.0 |
| Malta | 17.0 | 17.2 | 17.4 | 18.0 | 17.8 | 17.7 | 17.7 | 18.1 | 19.6 | 19.4 | 18.9 |
| Netherlands | 26.5 | 27.6 | 28.3 | 28.3 | 27.9 | 28.8 | 28.3 | 28.5 | 31.6 | 32.1 | 32.3 |
| Austria | 28.6 | 29.0 | 29.4 | 29.1 | 28.8 | 28.3 | 27.8 | 28.5 | 30.7 | 30.6 | 29.5 |
| Poland | 21.0 | 21.1 | 21.0 | 20.1 | 19.7 | 19.4 | 18.1 | 18.6 | 19.2 | 19.2 | 19.2 |
| Portugal | 21.9 | 22.8 | 23.2 | 23.8 | 24.5 | 24.5 | 23.9 | 24.3 | 26.8 | 26.8 | 26.5 |
| Romania | 12.8 | 13.6 | 13.1 | 12.8 | 13.4 | 12.8 | 13.6 | 14.3 | 17.1 | 17.6 | 16.3 |
| Slovenia | 24.4 | 24.3 | 23.6 | 23.3 | 23.0 | 22.7 | 21.3 | 21.4 | 24.2 | 25.0 | 25.0 |
| Slovakia | 18.9 | 19.1 | 18.4 | 17.2 | 16.5 | 16.4 | 16.1 | 16.1 | 18.8 | 187 | 18.2 |
| Finland | 25.0 | 25.7 | 26.6 | 26.7 | 26.7 | 26.4 | 25.4 | 26.2 | 30.4 | 30.6 | 30.0 |
| Sweden | 30.4 | 31.3 | 32.2 | 31.6 | 31.1 | 30.3 | 29.2 | 29.5 | 32.0 | 30.4 | 29.6 |
| United Kingdom | 26.6 | 25.6 | 25.5 | 25.7 | 25.8 | 25.6 | 24.7 | 25.8 | 28.6 | 27.4 | 27.3 |
| Iceland | 19.4 | 21.2 | 23.0 | 22.6 | 21.7 | 21.2 | 21.4 | 22.0 | 25.4 | 24.5 | 25.0 |
| Norway | 25.4 | 26.0 | 27.2 | 25.7 | 23.7 | 22.4 | 22.5 | 22.2 | 26.0 | 25.6 | 25.2 |
| Switzerland | 25.3 | 26.3 | 27.5 | 27.0 | 27.1 | 25.8 | 25.1 | 24.6 | 26.8 | 26.8 | 26.6 |
| Serbia | : | : | : | : | : | : | : | : | 24.6 | : | |

*Source:* Eurostat (online data code: spr_exp_sum) http://ec.europa.eu/eurostat/statistics-explained/index.php/Social_protection_statistics (accessed 18 January 2015).
*Note:* 1 = break in series.

the state in Northern Europe has actively worked to shape institutions and the labour market to produce more equal outcomes (Nuder 2012), the UK and the USA have followed a strategy of reducing or non-intervention and deregulation which has created enormous increases in inequality and destabilized economies. Over recent decades, some states, particularly the Nordic countries, have managed to resist growing

Table 2

Net replacement rates for six family types: initial phase of unemployment 2009, different earnings levels

| | 67% of average wage | | | | | | 100% of average wage | | | | | | 150% of average wage | | | | | |
| | No children | | | Two children | | | No children | | | Two children | | | No children | | | Two children | | |
| | | Married couple | | | Married couple | | | Married couple | | | Married couple | | | Married couple | | | Married couple | |
| | Single person | One-earner | Two-earner | Lone parent | One-earner | Two-earner | Single person | One-earner | Two-earner | Lone parent | One-earner | Two-earner | Single person | One-earner | Two-earner | Lone parent | One-earner | Two-earner |
|---|---|---|---|---|---|---|---|---|---|---|---|---|---|---|---|---|---|---|
| Denmark | 83 | 85 | 91 | 89 | 88 | 93 | 60 | 63 | 74 | 75 | 72 | 77 | 46 | 48 | 61 | 64 | 59 | 64 |
| Finland | 64 | 75 | 78 | 85 | 83 | 83 | 52 | 60 | 72 | 74 | 72 | 76 | 44 | 47 | 63 | 60 | 57 | 67 |
| Iceland | 77 | 72 | 89 | 84 | 77 | 91 | 77 | 80 | 86 | 83 | 83 | 88 | 56 | 61 | 71 | 65 | 67 | 74 |
| Ireland | 46 | 72 | 73 | 69 | 76 | 77 | 33 | 52 | 61 | 60 | 63 | 65 | 25 | 39 | 50 | 48 | 49 | 55 |
| Norway | 67 | 69 | 84 | 88 | 89 | 86 | 65 | 67 | 80 | 87 | 71 | 82 | 47 | 49 | 65 | 65 | 52 | 67 |
| Sweden | 69 | 69 | 85 | 83 | 80 | 86 | 48 | 48 | 69 | 65 | 58 | 71 | 36 | 36 | 58 | 51 | 44 | 60 |
| UK | 55 | 66 | 59 | 72 | 77 | 69 | 38 | 46 | 49 | 64 | 71 | 58 | 26 | 32 | 39 | 46 | 51 | 47 |

*Source*: OECD, Tax-benefit models, http://www.oecd.org/els/social/workincentives (accessed 16 January 2012).

Table 3

Unemployment Benefit replacement rates

World ranking in Unemployment Benefit replacement rates

| Country | Gross Replacement Rate, year 1 | Ranking | Country | Gross Replacement Rate, year 1 | Ranking |
|---------|-------------------------------|---------|---------|-------------------------------|---------|
| Netherlands | 0.7 | 1 | Egypt | 0.329 | 26 |
| Switzerland | 0.687 | 2 | Venezuela | 0.325 | 27 |
| Sweden | 0.685 | 3 | Belarus | 0.313 | 28 |
| Portugal | 0.65 | 4 | Israel | 0.307 | 29 |
| Spain | 0.635 | 5 | Japan | 0.289 | 30 |
| Norway | 0.624 | 6 | United States | 0.275 | 31 |
| Algeria | 0.612 | 7 | Kyrgyzstan | 0.255 | 32 |
| Taiwan | 0.6 | 8 | New Zealand | 0.254 | 33 |
| Ukraine | 0.56 | 9 | Latvia | 0.253 | 34 |
| Italy | 0.527 | 10 | India | 0.25 | 38 |
| Denmark | 0.521 | 11 | Korea, South | 0.25 | 37 |
| Russia | 0.505 | 12 | Uruguay | 0.25 | 36 |
| Tunisia | 0.5 | 13 | Uzbekistan | 0.25 | 35 |
| Finland | 0.494 | 14 | Ireland | 0.238 | 39 |
| France | 0.479 | 15 | Hungary | 0.235 | 40 |
| Bulgaria | 0.473 | 16 | Poland | 0.226 | 41 |
| Canada | 0.459 | 17 | Czech Republic | 0.225 | 42 |
| Romania | 0.45 | 18 | Australia | 0.21 | 43 |
| Hong Kong | 0.41 | 19 | Turkey | 0.206 | 44 |
| Austria | 0.398 | 20 | Albania | 0.202 | 45 |
| Belgium | 0.373 | 21 | United Kingdom | 0.189 | 46 |
| Argentina | 0.354 | 22 | Brazil | 0.152 | 47 |
| Germany | 0.353 | 23 | Estonia | 0.132 | 48 |
| Greece | 0.346 | 24 | Lithuania | 0.117 | 49 |
| Azerbaijan | 0.338 | 25 | Chile | 0.115 | 50 |
|  |  |  | Georgia | 0.09 | 51 |

*Source:* http://euwelfarestates.blogspot.co.uk/2012/04/world-ranking-in-unemployment-benefit.html (accessed 18 January 2015).

inequality by long-term policies of active labour market intervention (Wilkinson and Pickett 2009) and reasonable tax and social transfers. The Gini coefficient, a standard measure of income inequality that ranges from 0 (when everybody has identical incomes) to 1 (when all income goes to only one person), shows the UK to be one of the most unequal societies in the world, and inequality as a whole to be growing significantly over the past 30 years. Table 4 shows trends in real household income by income group, mid-1980s to late 2000s.

In the UK, while full-time earnings at the 90th percentile increased from £662 a week in 1984 to £1,007 a week in 2011, wages at the 10th

Figure 2

Gini coefficient of household disposable income and gap between richest
and poorest 10%, 2010

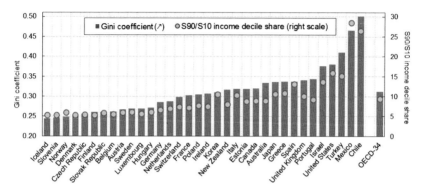

*Source:* https://makanaka.wordpress.com/tag/recession/ (accessed 18 January 2015).

percentile grew from just £218 to £279 over the same period. An implication of the incidence of low pay in the UK is that the labour share of gross domestic product (GDP) has become much more concentrated at the middle to top of the labour market. Amongst others (Bennett 2014), the Living Wage Commission has reported that:

> For the first time, the majority of people in poverty in the UK are working. One in every five workers are paid less than they need to maintain a basic, but socially acceptable standard of living. Working families are increasingly having to turn to food banks and credit to make ends meet (Living Wage Commission 2014: 6)

As well as the costs to the individual worker, low pay is a major cost to the public purse in terms of in-work benefits and additional social and other public services because poverty is linked to a range of problems

Table 4

Trends in real household income by income group, mid-1980s to late 2000s,
average annual percentage change

| Country | Total population | Top decile | Bottom decile |
|---------|------------------|------------|---------------|
| UK | 2.1 | 2.9 | 0.5 |

*Source:* An overview of growing income inequalities in OECD countries, http://www.oecd.org/els/soc/49499779.pdf (accessed 31 October 2014).

that the state has to address. For instance, between 2008 and 2013, real average income fell for Scots by 9.9 per cent (Nuder 2012). Kemp *et al.* (2013) have recorded how around a third of Local Housing Allowance claimant households contain someone in work, and this is higher in London where rents and housing costs generally are higher than in the country as a whole.

As the Organisation for Economic Co-operation and Development (OECD) has revealed (OECD 2011), across developed countries more and more wealth has been concentrating at the top and less and less has been trickling down. In its analysis it calls upon Atkinson (2009) to explain that this has been due to both growing earnings' shares at the top and declining shares at the bottom, but the highest earners have benefited especially (OECD 2011: 22). It continues by arguing that, 'Earners in the top 10% have been leaving the middle earners behind more rapidly than the lowest earners have been drifting away from the middle' (OECD 2011: 22). Now, only 12 pence of every pound of UK GDP goes to wages in the bottom half, down 25 per cent in the last three decades; and these trends have been more pronounced in the UK at both top and bottom than across the developed world (OECD 2011: table 1). Meanwhile, low pay is pervasive. One in five workers in Britain is paid below two-thirds of the median wage (below £7.49 an hour or £13,600 a year for full-time work) compared with fewer than one in ten in some other European countries (Neate 2013).

Using comparative and consistent data on poverty and low incomes from across the EU, it became apparent in the late 2000s that the UK was recording especially high levels of poverty (The Poverty Site 2011a). Those at 'risk of poverty or social exclusion' had reached the EU average by 2010 (UK: 23.1 per cent, compared with EU: 23.4 per cent), well in excess of all the Nordic countries, which varied between 14.3 and 18.3 per cent (CEC 2012a). As average incomes were higher across Northern Europe and inequality much lower, the composite position in the UK is appreciably worse in the UK than in these similar economies. More generally, this core set of poverty and social exclusion indicators have been regularly produced for every member state on a comparable basis and by 2009 showed that the UK had rates of poverty which were above the EU average and above the rates for all countries in northern and western Europe. Rates are particularly high relative to the average for children and those over 65 (The Poverty Site 2011b). For those in work, poverty was experienced at just below the EU average, but was worse for those unemployed; however, low income poverty was over a third and so higher than anywhere across the EU for the sick and disabled (The Poverty Site 2011c). This latter statistic is consistent with the Department for Work and Pensions' (DWP's) own time series which revealed an almost inexorable rise in rates of poverty of households with a disabled adult (DWP 2013) so that one-third were on low incomes compared with half that rate for all households.

As submitted to the Scottish Parliament in 2012, while the UK was comparable to most other developed and northern European economies up to the late 1970s, since then it has escalated throughout the intervening period before falling marginally and temporarily by 2010. Britain is now one of the most unequal and divided countries in the OECD and is returning to levels of inequity not seen since the 1930s (Lansley 2012). That relative change has not been inevitable but has been down to the choices made by successive UK governments (Sinfield 2011; Gulland 2014). The next section provides the theoretical underpinnings to analyze why this is harmful for both society and the economy.

## Literature Review and Theory

In its analysis of the impacts of rising inequality across the developed world, the OECD has concluded that:

> Rising income inequality creates economic, social and political challenges. It can stifle upward social mobility, making it harder for talented and hard-working people to get the rewards they deserve. Intergenerational earnings mobility is low in countries with high inequality such as Italy, the United Kingdom, and the United States, and much higher in the Nordic countries, where income is distributed more evenly (OECD, 2008). The resulting inequality of opportunity will inevitably impact economic performance as a whole (OECD 2011: 40)

In recent times, successful economies and societies have demonstrated high levels of coherence and equity, and an essential component in these performances has been the commitment to universalism. The Nordic countries in particular lead the world in terms of standards of living, innovation and creativity (CEC 2012b), equality and fairness (Sinfield 2011); their levels of benefits for those out of work or living with disabilities are close to average salaries and quality of life for all is prioritized (Danson 2012). This is consistent with the academic research which stresses partnership working and networking as the basis for economic competitiveness in the 21st century, rather than Fordist production models (Stiglitz 2012; Wilkinson and Pickett 2010). This emphasis on inclusion and involvement of workers, citizens and entrepreneurs with business and the state underpins the sustained high performances of these small nations and city regions in the Länder of Germany (Danson 2012). And key to these economic foundations are social contracts which promote identity with each other, the community and the nation through universalist principles.

In stark contrast are the so-called Anglo-Saxon welfare models of the USA and the UK. With their neo-liberal principles of competitiveness driving wages and benefits lower in real terms to try to achieve market share in low value added sectors of retailing and many services, they offer a vision of a society based on individualism and consumerism. The drivers invoked here promise rich rewards for a few and stagnation for

159

the many, as so cogently argued by commentators across the spectrum (see Elliott and Atkinson 2012, for their forecasts of how the UK's long-term decline will continue unabated into the future). In exploring neo-liberalism and the contemporary 'advanced liberal' rationality of government (Rose 1999), Barratt (2014: 266) discusses how 'advanced liberal rule seeks to promote the responsibility of individuals and collectivities for determining their own fate (Rose 1999)'. In particular, Barratt notes that in 'the promotion of social welfare ... the unemployed subject is increasingly responsible for his or her own self-government as an active jobseeker', but this freedom to act is regulated by an array of governmental forces including think tank intellectuals and jobcentre and DWP managers who 'monitor and scrutinize his or her conduct on a daily basis' (Barratt 2014: 266), Van Gerven and Ossewaarde (2012) offer similar arguments in these respects. In brief, universalism and the very concept of certain universal benefits being available to all have come under extreme attack in the last two decades as the post-war Keynesian consensus has been destroyed.

In the second section of this article on 'Comparative Analyses', many of the statistics were sourced from 2011 or earlier. This was for two reasons: the delays and revisions to many such statistics mean that a cautious approach is sensible and, second, the financial crisis and subsequent austerity measures introduced by the coalition Government had not yet taken full hold on relative incomes and poverty. This latter point is important as the trends and positions of the poor and those on social security benefits were still dominated by decisions and policies applied during the long period of growth in the UK economy. There is further complementary evidence on the progressive embedding of the differing, more punitive welfare approach in Britain; for example, Van Gerven and Ossewaarde (2012: 51), based on their international comparisons, have argued that 'The British welfare state appears to have been most radical in the individualization of social rights'. The statistics and reports cited here therefore reflect how the UK now treats its most vulnerable during times of prosperity, and it is all too apparent that the UK is currently but half way through a decade of cuts and austerity measures which are impacting most severely on those on low incomes (McKendrick *et al.* 2014; Goulden 2012; Trebeck 2013).

Social contracts, universalist principles and the promotion of mutual identification are significant, therefore, in reinforcing the drivers, motivations, values and norms that underpin different national approaches. These are critical to understanding differences in public attitudes and, ultimately, national welfare regimes, but at present these remain underdeveloped in the wider literature on welfare regimes, partly because of a relative lack of data and intelligence gathered on a consistent basis (Blekesaune and Quadagno 2003). The secondary data presented here are similarly limited and restrict the capacity to explore these issues in any detail. However, in an early attempt to understand national (as opposed to individuals') differences in attitudes towards welfare state policies, Blekesaune and Quadagno (2003) concluded that 'egalitarian nations' have more positive public attitudes on policies for the unemployed, but there were fewer differences with regard to the sick and the old. They suggested that:

> nations generate different public beliefs about national social problems and about the relationship between individuals, the state and other institutions. Eventually, these understandings and beliefs influence popular attitudes regarding what kind of policies the state should pursue, and who should benefit (Blekesaune and Quadagno 2003: 415)

Examined in the context of other countries' approaches to active labour market policies (ALMPs), it has been argued that many elements of the welfare regime in the UK are self-defeating and contradictory with penalties and conditions reducing the agency or ability of those on benefits to act (Bennett 2014; Wright 2012). The demonization of the poor, promoted through the media (for specific examples, see Trebeck 2012; Wynne-Jones n.d.a; for further critiques, see Wynne-Jones n.d.b), is long-established in the UK (Gulland 2014), and Spicker (2014a) has analyzed some of the continuing myths about the poor.

It has been proposed[1] that, given these data and conceptual challenges, there is merit in exploring whether the processes of identification (De Swaan 1995, 1997; Jenkins 2004) might underpin these ideological differences. There have been studies into how 'the state/elites mobilize these disidentifications in legitimizing neoliberal policies of welfare retrenchment (Slater 2013); and how national habitus (i.e. norms and values), developed over the very long-term helps explain differences in welfare attitudes between nations (De Swaan 1988)'.[1] The insights by De Swann in particular are based on research in zones of extreme conflict but offer an opportunity for entry into the use of populism by neo-liberal regimes regarding social security claimants, 'At the base of this operation seems to be a coalition of agents, in a certain way referable to the middle class, determined to create their social antagonists by building up an artificial opposition between "Hutu" and "Tutsi" '.

The references above to divisive and populist[2] media reports question why Britain (and the British public) is less willing to provide support for those on welfare than Benelux and Nordic countries. The research by Blekesaune and Quadagno (2003) appears to take the understanding some way further, although there remains a certain degree of tautology in applying their findings.

In the latest publication on the position of the poor specifically in Scotland, *Poverty in Scotland 2014*, McKendrick *et al.* (2014) describe the deteriorating status of those dependent on social security since 2010 – whether or not they are in work. In that edited collection, the comparative chapters on social security and welfare systems in other parts of Europe and beyond are both sober assessments of differences and failings, but also of the norms and values that underpin different national approaches. It is striking that the systems in the Nordic countries and the Basque country are introduced in terms of their contribution to 'solidarity', 'inclusion' and 'cohesion'. These are the same terms that are believed to drive the superior economic development performances of these small nation states according to both academic literature and policy prescriptions at national, European and supranational organizational levels.

So, applying concepts associated with Martin, it can be argued that these nations on the periphery of the EU have shown degrees of resilience since the financial crisis started that suggests that their cohesion and flexibility have much to offer as models for resistance and success (Martin 2010).

Endogenous growth and smart specialization have become key strategic approaches to economic development, and each is based on building social capital, networks and partnerships between enterprises, government and community (Landabosa 2012; Camagni and Capello 2012; Morgan and Nauwelaers 1999; Roseta-Palma *et al.* 2010). They rely on proximity, trust and tacit knowledge (Ferri *et al.* 2009), and Knack and Keefer (1997: 1251) provide:

> evidence that 'social capital' matters for measurable economic performance, using indicators of trust and civic norms ... [which] We find ... are stronger in nations with higher and more equal incomes, with institutions that restrain predatory actions of chief executives, and with better-educated and ethnically homogeneous populations.

The most successful economies and societies in global league tables are characterized by low levels of inequality, high levels of gender equality and press freedom, and high degrees of happiness and life-satisfaction (table 5; Danson 2012). They also have the most inclusive and 'generous' (Sinfield 2011) social security systems; it is argued below that these are not unrelated and the causality is mutually reinforcing.

## Policy Choices and Contexts

From their composite index of health and social problems (which incorporates indicators of 'Life expectancy, Math & Literacy, Infant mortality, Homicides, Imprisonment, Teenage births, Trust, Obesity, Mental illness – including: drug & alcohol, addiction, and Social mobility'), Wilkinson and Pickett (2009) confirm the strong correlation between higher levels of equality and better records on this multidimensional scale. The construction of the Oxfam Humankind index (Oxfam Scotland 2013) has revealed the consensus around what are considered across society as being the significant basic elements of a good life and society: good health, a home to live in, meaningful work or activity, a

Table 5

Select comparison of international social justice and competitiveness measures

| Country | UNHDI ranking (2012)[1] | Gini coefficient (2010)[2] Higher value indicates greater inequality | World Bank ease of doing business (2014)[3] | IMD competitiveness (2013)[4] | WEF competitiveness (2013–14)[5] |
|---|---|---|---|---|---|
| Denmark | 15 | 0.252 | 5 | 12 | 15 |
| Finland | 21 | 0.26 | 12 | 20 | 3 |
| Ireland | 7 | 0.331 | 15 | 17 | 28 |
| New Zealand | 6 | 0.317 | 3 | 25 | 18 |
| Norway | 1 | 0.249 | 9 | 6 | 11 |
| Sweden | 7 | 0.269 | 14 | 4 | 6 |
| Switzerland | 9 | 0.298 | 29 | 2 | 1 |
| UK | 26 | 0.341 | 10 | 18 | 10 |

*Notes:* 1 = United Nations Human Development Index, 2012 (Scottish Government 2013), OECD and other references embedded into this source; 2 = OECD Statistics, http://www.oecd.org/social/inequality.htm (accessed 31 October 2014); 3 = *Doing Business 2014*, World Bank, 29 October 2013; 4 = IMD *World Competitiveness Yearbook*, May 2013; 5 = *Global Competitiveness Report 2013–2014*, World Economic Forum, September 2013.

degree of status and respect of peers, and security or reduction of anxiety and fear in respect to having and keeping these things. These elements are deeply interconnected. 'A good society would be a social and economic system that made sure everyone has the best chance of achieving this rounded understanding of Social Security' (McKay and Sullivan 2014: 4).

In keeping with the approach that seeks to improve living standards and so promote economic performance without adversely affecting incentives and the costs to the state, the widespread adoption of a 'living wage' has been encouraged as an extension of the rationale behind the minimum wage. A report for the Trades Union Congress by Howard Reed of Landman Economics (TUC 2013) has estimated that £246.4 million of savings could be made by the public purse in Scotland if the 416,000 workers currently earning below the living wage (£7.45 per hour at the time of the analysis) received the living wage. The Government would receive an extra £161.7 million from the increased tax and national insurance contributions (NIC) and would pay out £84.7 million less in means-tested benefits and tax credits. These figures factor in the effects of income tax, NIC, tax credits and other means tested benefits. Across the UK, that same analysis estimated the Treasury would gain an extra £2.1 billion from the increased NIC if the living wage was applied nationally at current rates of £8.55 an hour in London and £7.45 elsewhere in the UK. Also, in-work means-tested benefits and tax credits would be reduced saving the Treasury £1.1 billion; leading to improvements in the state budget of £3.2 billion.

As well as suppressing family incomes and local spending, low levels of benefits and poor pay do not offer the incentives and rewards for many careers that are meant to underpin the Anglo-Saxon welfare model. Recent research on the Scottish labour market has confirmed that there are ongoing failures in the utilization and application of skills in the economy, to the inevitable detriment of enterprises, workers and society overall (Keep 2013). While the nations and regions of the UK have long suffered from the loss of talent and expertize to the labour market escalator of London and the South East to the long-term cost of their respective economies (Fielding 1992; Danson 2005), these newer failures have been exacerbating the rigidities and constraints to mobility more generally. Inflated house prices and other congestion externalities have made it difficult for migrant workers to move to this region and so to realize their potential in the labour market or career (see BBC 2014, based on reports by Civitas and Ernst Young; Kemp *et al.* 2013). In a market-dependent social security system, where individual movement to find work or promotion to maximize returns is a critical driver and presumption of effective and efficient labour and housing markets is fundamental to the expected successes of its operations, Germany offers a better model. As McKay and Sullivan (2014: 12–13) argue, 'If we had Germany's levels of house price stability and therefore rent stability this would be a huge advantage in savings and planning for a welfare budget'.

On mobility more broadly, Wilkinson and Pickett have revealed the emphatic negative correlation between social mobility and income inequality (Wilkinson and Pickett 2010: 22); in virtuous and vicious cycles of causation, forces for mobility and equality interact across many dimensions to generate more beneficial outcomes for the common good. This reinforcement of negative relationships between key drivers and variables in the economy at both the individual and aggregate levels undermines the capacity of the social security system in the UK to achieve its narrow objectives discussed earlier. The reliance on market mechanisms to ensure the operations of the welfare system fulfil their obligations to eradicate poverty and promote economic efficiency are undermined and indeed countered by the market failures endemic in this country.

Within the context of the long run increase in inequality in the UK and the USA, and the dissemination of this tendency to other countries, the OECD has argued that policies for redistribution are key to reversing polarization and improving economic performance (OECD 2011). In summary: 'Reforming tax and benefit policies is the most direct and powerful instrument for increasing redistributive effects' (OECD 2011: 40). Because of tax and benefit constraints, the rise of populism and other macro-economic factors, more and better jobs are seen as crucial in addressing endemic poverty and inequality, as argued by both the OECD and the Jimmy Reid Foundation

(2013) in Scotland. They directly link the nature of work with positive change:

> Recent trends towards higher rates of in-work poverty indicate that job quality has become a concern for a growing number of workers. Policy reforms that tackle inequalities in the labour market, such as those between standard and non-standard forms of employment, are needed to reduce income inequality (OECD 2011: 41)

While in its Common Weal papers the Jimmy Reid Foundation has argued for an essential role for collective bargaining (Duffy *et al.* 2013; Koeninger *et al.* 2007; Visser and Cecchi 2009; Cecchi and García-Peñalosa 2008) to complement wider fiscal and employment legislation:

> security of employment and security of income from employment will require a different approach to industrial democracy. A strong and constructive relationship between trade unions and employers with the assumption of widespread collective bargaining and strong employment rights is an essential foundation for ensuring that work pays and that the welfare state is not required to pick up the cost of employment practices that lead to poverty (McKay and Sullivan 2014: 11)

## Reforming Social Security: A Citizen's Basic Income

In promoting the lessons from the Swedish recovery from economic recession in the early 1990s, Per Nuder, the former Swedish finance minister, has argued along similar lines to the OECD (2011) on what works. He suggests:

- The Swedish approach was based on clear value, underpinned by the 'Swedish model', which incorporates such priorities as lifelong learning, protecting people not jobs, and the importance of ALMPs.
- Pro-employment policies were future-focused, based on a long-term analysis of what the economy would look like after the recession.
- The politics of budget-balancing and labour market reform were attached to a broader vision, proving that the Swedish model was not dead and turning the fight against unemployment into a national project. (Nuder 2012)

In the foregoing, this article argues that, while some of these elements are in place in the UK and in Scotland in particular, the transformation of the social security system from an Anglo-Saxon welfare state into a more Nordic model is required (McKay and Sullivan 2014). In a virtuous cycle of better jobs leading to higher household incomes for those at the bottom resulting in higher local and national activity and value added, this would allow the improvements in economic performance necessary to fund more inclusive and efficient social security.

At present, the benefit system in the UK as configured is incredibly complicated (McKay and Sullivan 2014: 16). It is therefore inefficient as claimants and advisers are increasingly unable to predict reasonably the effects and outcomes, especially in terms of its interaction with the tax system. That presents labour market issues and further inefficiencies so that simplification would not only make integration possible but also make the whole system more efficient. A significant problem with the current benefit system is its interaction with its various elements and with the tax system so as to produce anomalies and unintended consequences, such as penalties for taking small infrequent pieces of work, part-time work or starting a business. Rapid withdrawals of benefits and high levels of tax on initial earnings are well documented. The new Universal Credit seeks to tackle some of these issues. There are of course a number of additional problems with the Universal Credit (Brewer *et al.* 2012; Spicker 2014b) which make a Citizens' income a much better solution to these problems, whilst also removing benefits' stigma and providing wider social and economic benefits. The idea of a Citizens' Income or Citizen's Basic Income (CBI) has been around for a long time now and has been well researched and documented, including a number of successful pilot programmes in different parts of the world (Atkinson 1996; De Wispelaere and Noguera 2012; Fisher and Gilbert 2014; McKay 2005; Torry 2013; Yanes 2012).

The CBI would be a tax-free cash transfer made to every citizen probably on a monthly basis. This would be a basic amount on which every citizen can survive excluding housing and any extra costs for disability living. One model is for the rate to be variable by age so families with children get a payment for each child and older people get a basic state pension. It is necessary to have a separate housing benefit linked with an overall housing strategy and an equality/care benefit linked with social care policy as detailed above. This is a way of providing a safety net for all and provide a platform from which people will be incentivized to work in order to have extra income on top of the basic and to save money without penalty. Evidence from a pilot in Dauphin, Manitoba and from analogous experiments in the global south and elsewhere suggest that some of the problems that have been claimed would arise from unconditional direct money transfers do not transpire (McKay and Sullivan 2014: 16–17). It seems it is rarely misspent and does not disincentivize work.

In her *post hoc* evaluation of the Dauphin experiment, Forget identifies a series of positive social and economic outcomes which have persisted (Forget 2011). The OECD has recorded the advantages of a CBI more comprehensively:

1. households make good use of the money;
2. poverty decreases;
3. long-term benefits in income, health and tax income are remarkable;

4. there is no negative effect on labour supply – recipients do not work less; and
5. the programmes save money (Barrientos and Hulme 2010).

These evaluations conclude that it seems unconditional income stimulates the entire economy: consumption goes up, resulting in more jobs and higher incomes.

Modelling supports this also, with Colombino *et al.* (2009) agreeing that 'universal basic income is optimal' in addressing the standard challenges in social security and welfare issues: as McKay and Sullivan (2014) argue these include 'simplification and rationalization of redistributive policies' (drawing on Friedman and Tobin); similarly, both teams also refer to 'Flexicurity' (income – rather than job – stability and certainty); and 'efficiency'. Interestingly, the final essential factor in all the rationales encompasses a 'dividend' from the 'Common' or the 'Social Capital' echoing the Common Weal origins of the Jimmy Reid Foundation (2013) approach.

As a contribution to the debate on how radical changes to the social security system could support improvements in the economic performance of Scotland, as an exemplar for other parts of the UK, McKay and Sullivan have provided a worked example of a CBI. Their particular scheme is funded by removing tax allowances and relief and phasing out means-tested and contributory benefits. In addition, Income Tax and employees' NICs could be merged into a new Income Tax. The scheme could be derived from a high pay, high employment economy and a reformed tax system as detailed in a companion paper 'Investing in the Good Society' (Danson *et al.* 2013) and savings made through increased revenue and reduced in-work benefits estimated at £246.4 million. The CBI scheme outlined is close to being revenue-and cost-neutral.

As a key element of building an integrated tax and benefit system which promotes coherence and inclusion, a CBI presents a means of complementing the other parts of Sweden's programme for recovery which has gone on to sustain through two further decades.

## Conclusions

In this article, it is shown that successful economies and societies are based on social security systems which are based on values and norms of inclusion, cohesion and coherence. These lead to high wage economies with high value-added activities in the economy promoting high national economic performance. Such economies have shown resilience during downturns and recessions with stability and fairness complements.

By contrast, the UK presents itself to the world as a highly unequal, low wage, divided and debt-ridden country apparently destined to underperform economically in a seemingly inexorable path to decline; or, as described in the title of the recent book by Elliott and Atkinson (2012), *Going South: Why Britain will have a Third World Economy by 2014.* Further

167

research is required to determine whether there are particular features in the UK of (dis)identifications and resultant stigma (Blekesaune and Quadagno 2003) and how these inform policy, for example both policies towards Roma across Europe as well as welfare recipients, and some of the other contributions to this Special Issue serve this agenda to an extent. Another way of approaching this would be through the British Social Attitudes survey time-series data (using the questions on attitudes to welfare).

By contrast with the UK, some of the countries which are closest neighbours enjoy appreciable higher levels of performance and living standards. Indeed, we have argued elsewhere (Danson 2014: 188) that:

> On virtually every possible measure of social and economic success, all league tables are topped by societies with strong universal welfare states (Danson 2012). Because they have these universal social contracts they are high performers; it is not because they can afford them that they are able to have generous systems, but it is the reverse that is critical – inclusion and cohesion are the fundamentals for success (Stiglitz 2012; Wilkinson and Pickett 2009)

Here, we argue that our economy and society must be considered as an integrated whole – integrated and multi-dimensional. In effect, all of us create our society and shape our environment. That building and shaping and thinking, and creating can be defined in one word – work. The role of the state is to create a system where that effort citizens put into work creates the society we want. As in the neoliberal Anglo-Saxon system of social security and the Nordic and similar welfare states, central to the Common Weal vision and to its approach to welfare is the idea of work. In the Nordic countries it is taken for granted that a high level of welfare is achieved through high standards of work. A political economy that delivered solidarity and high levels of employment with good wages would be better able to afford a welfare system that achieves 'social security'. As argued here, as it would be based on foundations of cohesion, inclusion and coherence, it would also promise to deliver higher levels of economic individual and societal prosperity and performance (The Jimmy Reid Foundation 2013). A CBI has been proposed as overcoming many of the constraints and adverse effects of the current welfare system while also preserving incentives for individual and social investment in human and social capital.

## Acknowledgements

This article is dedicated to Professor Ailsa McKay, co-author, who died only a few days after completing some of the key arguments incorporated here (and discussed in McKay and Sullivan 2014). Professor of economics at Glasgow Caledonian University, Ailsa was a passionate advocate of a welfare system that created security in the place of anxiety and of a CBI to ensure all members of society have that security. We hope that part of her legacy will be a national approach to welfare which lives up to her ideals.

## Notes

* Corresponding author.
1. We are very grateful to an anonymous referee for the suggestion to explore 'disidentification' in addressing the limitations in the data and literature; this has benefited the article significantly but any errors in interpretation should not be laid at the referee's door.
2. An ideology that 'pits a virtuous and homogeneous people against a set of elites and dangerous "others" who were together depicted as depriving (or attempting to deprive) the sovereign people of their rights, values, prosperity, identity, and voice' (Albertazzi and McDonnell 2008: 3).

## References

Albertazzi, D. and McDonnell, D. (2008), *Twenty-First Century Populism: The Spectre of Western European Democracy*, Basingstoke: Palgrave Macmillan.

Atkinson, A. B. (1996), The case for a participation income, *The Political Quarterly*, 67, 1: 67–70.

Atkinson, A. B. (2009), *The Changing Distribution of Earnings in OECD Countries*, Oxford: Oxford University Press.

Barratt, E. (2014), Bureaucracy, citizenship, governmentality: towards a re-evaluation of New Labour, *Ephemera: Theory and Politics in Organization*, 14, 2: 263–80.

Barrientos, A. and Hulme, D. (2010), *Just Give Money to the Poor: The Development Revolution from the Global South*, Manchester: Brooks World Poverty Institute, University of Manchester, http://www.oecd.org/dev/pgd/46240619.pdf (accessed 31 October 2014).

BBC (2014), Housing bubble forming in London, http://www.bbc.co.uk/news/business-26006214 (accessed 12 April 2014).

Bennett, H. (2014), The short-sightedness of 'poverty punishment' tools in Active Labour Market Policies, http://challengepoverty.wordpress.com/2014/10/16/the-short-sightedness-of-poverty-punishment-tools-in-active-labour-market-policies/ (accessed 31 October 2014).

Blekesaune, M. and Quadagno, J. (2003), Public attitudes toward welfare state policies: a comparative analysis of 24 nations, *European Sociological Review*, 19, 5: 415–27.

Brady, D. (2009), *Rich Democracies Poor Societies: How Politics Explain Poverty*, Oxford: Oxford University Press.

Brewer, M., Browne, J. and Wenchao, J. (2012), Universal Credit: a preliminary analysis of its impact on incomes and work incentives, *Fiscal Studies*, 33, 1: 39–71.

Camagni, R. and Capello, R. (2012), *Regional innovation patterns and the EU regional policy reform: towards smart innovation policies*, Paper given at the 52nd ERSA Conference, Bratislava, Slovakia, 21–24 August.

CEC (2012a), At risk of poverty or social exclusion, Eurostat press release 21/2012 – 8 February, http://ec.europa.eu/eurostat/web/products-press-releases/-/3-08022012-AP (accessed 18 January 2015).

CEC (2012b), Industrial innovation: Innovation Union Scoreboard, European Commission website, http://ec.europa.eu/enterprise/policies/innovation/files/ius-2011_en.pdf (accessed 18 January 2015).

Cecchi, D. and García-Peñalosa, C. (2008), *Labour Market Institutions and the Personal Distribution of Income in the OECD*, Document de Travail 2008-47, GREQAM. http:// hal.inria.fr/docs/00/34/10/05/PDF/DI2008-47.pdf (accessed 31 October 2014).

Colombino, U., Locatelli, M., Narazani, E. and Shima, I. (2009), *Behavioural and Welfare Effects of Basic Income Schemes*, http://www.frdb.org/upload/file/presentation_81107_colombino.pdf (accessed 31 October 2014).

Danson, M. (2005), Old industrial regions and employability, *Urban Studies*, 42, 2: 285–300.

Danson, M. (2012), *Whose economy? Scotland in Northern Europe: balancing dynamic economies with greater social equality*, Paper given at the Scottish Parliament Economy, Energy and Tourism Committee 4th annual joint seminar with the STUC on 'Growth versus the Scottish Government's "Golden Rules" and Economic Strategy', Edinburgh, UK, 21 February, http://www.scottish.parliament.uk/parliamentarybusiness/CurrentCommittees/47772.aspx (accessed 31 October 2014).

Danson, M. (2014), The benefits of universalism. In J. H. McKendrick, G. Mooney, J. Dickie, G. Scott and P. Kelly (eds), *Poverty in Scotland 2014: The Independence Referendum and Beyond*, London: Child Poverty Action Group.

Danson, M. and Trebeck, K. (2013), *No More Excuses: How a Common Weal Approach Can End Poverty in Scotland*, Glasgow: The Jimmy Reid Foundation.

Danson, M., Macfarlane, L. and Sullivan, W. (2013), *Investing in the Good Society. Five questions on Tax and the Common Weal*, Glasgow: The Jimmy Reid Foundation.

Danson, M., McAlpine, R., Spicker, P. and Sullivan, W. (2012), *The Case for Universalism. An Assessment of the Evidence on the Effectiveness and Efficiency of the Universal Welfare State*, Glasgow: The Jimmy Reid Foundation.

Department for Work and Pensions (DWP) (2013), *Households Below Average Income. An analysis of the income distribution 1994/95–2011/12*, London: DWP, https://www.gov.uk/government/uploads/system/uploads/attachment_data/file/206778/full_hbai13.pdf (accessed 18 April 2014).

De Swaan, A. (1988), *In Care of the State: Health Care, Education and Welfare in Europe and the USA in the Modern Era*, Cambridge: Polity Press.

De Swaan, A. (1995), Widening circles of identification: emotional concerns in socio-genetic perspective, *Theory, Culture and Society*, 12, 1: 25–39.

De Swaan, A. (1997), Widening circles of disidentification: on the psycho- and socio-genesis of the hatred of distant strangers – reflections on Rwanda, *Theory, Culture and Society*, 4, 2: 105–22.

De Wispelaere, J. and Noguera, J. A. (2012), On the political feasibility of universal basic income: an analytic framework. In R. Caputo (ed.), *Basic Income Guarantee and Politics: International Experiences and Perspectives on the Viability of Income Guarantee*, New York, NY: Palgrave Macmillan, pp. 17–38.

Duffy, J., Gall, G. and Mather, J. (2013), *Working Together: A Vision for Industrial Democracy in a Common Weal Economy*, Glasgow: The Jimmy Reid Foundation.

Elliott, L. and Atkinson, D. (2012), *Going South: Why Britain Will Have a Third World Economy by 2014*, London: Palgrave Macmillan.

European Commission (2013), Social protection per inhabitant, http://epp.eurostat.ec.europa.eu/statistics_explained/index.php/Social_protection_statistics (accessed 31 October 2014).

Ferri, P., Deakins, D. and Whittam, G. (2009), The measurement of social capital in the entrepreneurial context, *Journal of Enterprising Communities: People and Places in the Global Economy*, 3, 2: 138–51.

Fielding, A. J. (1992), Migration and social mobility: South East England as an 'escalator' region, *Regional Studies*, 26, 1: 1–15.

Fisher, M. and Gilbert, J. (2014), *Reclaim Modernity. Beyond Markets, Beyond Machines*, http://compass.3cdn.net/614d8d010cb4b4d88f_f5m6br746.pdf (accessed 31 October 2014).

Forget, E. (2011), Research profile – Life in a town without poverty, http://www.saskdisc.ca/2011/07/research-profile-life-in-a-town-without-poverty-research-article-of-interest/ (accessed 11 April 2014).

Goulden, C. (2012), The relentless rise of in-work poverty, JRF Blog, http://www.jrf.org.uk/blog/2012/06/relentless-rise-work-poverty (accessed 31 October 2014).

Gulland, J. (2014), Poverty and disability benefits: a view from the past, http://challengepoverty.wordpress.com/2014/10/13/poverty-and-disability-benefits-a-view-from-the-past/ (accessed 31 October 2014).

Hunter, L., Senior, G., Danson, M., Jardine, A. and Sym, L. (1988), *Information Gaps in the Local Labour Market*, Aldershot: Avebury.

Jenkins, R. (2004), *Social Identity*, 2nd edn, London: Routledge.

Jimmy Reid Foundation, The (2013), *The Common Weal: A Model for Economic and Social Development in Scotland*, Glasgow: The Jimmy Reid Foundation.

Keep, E. (2013), *Opening the 'Black Box' – The Increasing Importance of a Public Policy Focus on What Happens in the Workplace, Skills in Focus*, Glasgow: Skills Development Scotland.

Kemp, P., Hall, S. and Pereira, I. (2013), *The Early Impacts of the LHA Reforms on the Experiences and Perceptions of LHA Claimants: Monitoring the Impact of Changes to the Local Housing Allowance System of Housing Benefit: Interim Report*, London: Department for Work and Pensions.

Knack, S. and Keefer, P. (1997), Does social capital have an economic payoff? A cross-country investigation, *The Quarterly Journal of Economics*, 112, 4: 1251–88.

Koeninger, W., Leonardi, M. and Nunziata, L. (2007), Labour market institutions and wage inequality, *Industrial & Labor Relations Review*, 60, 3: 340–56.

Lamont, J. (2012), Labour leader Johann Lamont demands end to 'something for nothing' culture, http://news.stv.tv/politics/191807-labour-leader-johann-lamont-demands-end-to-something-for-nothing-culture/ (accessed 31 October 2014).

Landabosa, M. (2012), *Research and Innovation Strategies for Smart Specialization*, Presentation to the OECD, Paris, France, 19 June, http://www.oecd.org/dev/ 50649698.pdf (accessed 31 October 2014).

Lansley, S. (2012), *Inequality, the 2008 Crash and the Ongoing Crisis*, Paper given at the Scottish Parliament Economy, Energy and Tourism Committee 4th annual joint seminar with the STUC on 'Growth versus the Scottish Government's "Golden Rules" and Economic Strategy', Edinburgh, UK, 21 February, http://www.scottish.parliament.uk/parliamentarybusiness/CurrentCommittees/47772.aspx (accessed 31 October 2014).

Living Wage Commission (2014), *Working for Poverty. The Scale of the Problem of Low Pay and Working Poverty in the UK*, London: Living Wage Commission.

Martin, R. (2010), Regional economic resilience, hysteresis and recessionary shocks, *Journal of Economic Geography*, 12, 1: 1–32.

McKay, A. (2005), *The Future of Social Security Policy: Women, Work and a Citizen's Basic Income*, London: Routledge.

McKay, A. and Sullivan, W. (2014), *In Place of Anxiety: Social Security for the Common Weal*, Biggar: Reid Foundation and Compass.

McKendrick, J. H., Mooney, G., Dickie, J., Scott, G. and Kelly, P. (eds) (2014), *Poverty in Scotland 2014: The Independence Referendum and Beyond*, London: Child Poverty Action Group.

Mooney, G. (2014), Poverty, 'austerity' and Scotland's constitutional future. In J. H. McKendrick, G. Mooney, J. Dickie, G. Scott and P. Kelly (eds), *Poverty in Scotland 2014: The Independence Referendum and Beyond*, London: Child Poverty Action Group, pp. 3–27.

Morgan, K. and C. Nauwelaers (1999), A regional perspective on innovation: from theory to strategy. In K. Morgan and C. Nauwelaers (eds), *Regional Innovation Strategies: The Challenge for Less-Favoured Regions*, London: The Stationery Office and Regional Studies Association, pp. 9–24.

Neate, R. (2013), Pay workers more, CBI chief tells thriving firms, *Guardian* 30 December, http://www.theguardian.com/money/2013/dec/30/pay-workers-more-cbi-firms (accessed 31 October 2014).

Nuder, P. (2012), *Saving the Swedish Model: Learning from Sweden's Return to Full Employment in the Late 1990s*, London: Institute for Public Policy Research.

Organisation for Economic Co-operation and Development (OECD) (2008), *Growing Unequal? Income Distribution in OECD Countries*, Paris: OECD.

Organisation for Economic Co-operation and Development (OECD) (2011), *Divided We Stand: Why Inequality Keeps Rising*, Paris: OECD.

Oxfam Scotland (2013), The *Oxfam Humankind Index: The New Measure of Scotland's Prosperity*, http://policy-practice.oxfam.org.uk/our-work/poverty-in-the-uk/humankind-index (accessed 31 October 2014).

Poverty Site, The (2011a), http://www.poverty.org.uk/index.htm (accessed 31 October 2014).

Poverty Site, The (2011b), *Low Income by Age and Gender*, http://www.poverty.org.uk/e01a/index.shtml (accessed 31 October 2014).

Poverty Site, The (2011c), *Low Income and Disability*, http://www.poverty.org.uk/40/index.shtml?2 (accessed 31 October 2014).

Rose, N. (1999), *Powers of Freedom: Reclaiming Political Thought*, Cambridge: Cambridge University Press.

Roseta-Palma, C., Lopes, A. and Sequeira, T. N. (2010), Externalities in an endogenous growth model with social and natural capital, *Ecological Economics*, 69, 3: 603–12.

Salmond, A. (2013), *Addressing Alienation – The Opportunity of Independence*, Jimmy Reid Foundation Lecture, Govan, UK, 29 January, https://www.snp.org/blog/post/2013/jan/first-ministers-jimmy-reid-foundation-lecture (accessed 31 October 2014).

Scottish Government (2013), *Building Security and Creating Opportunity: Economic Policy Choices in an Independent Scotland*, Edinburgh: Scottish Government, http://www.scotland.gov.uk/Publications/2013/11/2439/5 (accessed 31 October 2014).

Sinfield, A. (2011), *Whose Welfare State Now?, A Whose Economy? Seminar Paper*, Oxford: Oxfam.

Slater, T. (2013), The myth of 'Broken Britain': welfare reform and the production of ignorance, *Antipode*, 45, 1: 1–22.

Spicker, P. (2014a), *A Few Myths about Poverty*, http://challengepoverty.wordpress.com/2014/10/13/a-few-myths-about-poverty/ (accessed 31 October 2014).

Spicker, P. (2014b), Universal Credit: don't blame the IT, *Computer Weekly*, http://www.computerweekly.com/opinion/Universal-Credit-Dont-blame-the-IT (accessed 11 April 2014).

Stiglitz, J. (2012), *The Price of Inequality: How Today's Divided Society Endangers Our Future*, New York, NY: WW Norton.

Torry, M. (2013), *Money for Everyone: Why We Need a Citizen's Income*, Bristol: Policy Press.

Trades Union Congress (TUC) (2013), *Paying the Living Wage would Mean a £3.2 billion Boost to Public Finances*, http://www.tuc.org.uk/economic-issues/britain-needs-pay-rize/economic-analysis/paying-living-wage-would-mean-%C2%A332-billion (accessed 11 April 2014).

Trebeck, K. (2012), *Conspicuously Poor*, http://www.oxfam.org.uk/get-involved/campaign-with-us/latest-campaign-news/2012/01/conspicuously-poor?cid=aff_affwd (accessed 31 October 2014).

Trebeck, K. (2013), *Our Economy: Towards a New Prosperity*, Oxford: Oxfam GB, http:// policypractice.oxfam.org.uk/publications/our-economy-towards-a-new-prosperity -294239 (accessed 18 January 2015).

Van Gerven, M. and Ossewaarde, M. (2012), The welfare state's making of cosmopolitan Europe: individualization of social rights as European integration, *European Societies*, 14, 1: 35–55.

Visser, J. and Cecchi, D. (2009), Inequality and the labour market: unions. In W. Salverda, B. Nolan and T. Smeeding (eds), *Oxford Handbook of Economic Inequality*, Oxford: Oxford University Press, pp. 230–56.

Wilkinson, R. and Pickett, K. (2009), *The Spirit Level: Why Equality is Better for Everyone*, Harmondsworth: Penguin.

Wilkinson, R. and Pickett, K. (2010), *The Spirit Level: Why Equality is Better for Everyone*, Guest Lecture given at the Wolfson Research Institute, Durham University, England, UK, 12 March.

Wright, S. (2012), Welfare-to-work, agency and personal responsibility, *Journal of Social Policy*, 41, 2: 309–28.

Wynne-Jones, R. (n.d.a), *Deserving vs Undeserving*, http://www.jrf.org.uk/reporting-poverty/journalists-experiences/deserving-undeserving (accessed 31 October 2014).

Wynne-Jones, R. (n.d.b), *Journalists' Experiences: 'We need to report poverty in all its ugliness, yet without exploiting it'*, http://www.jrf.org.uk/reporting-poverty/journalists-experiences (accessed 31 October 2014).

Yanes, P. (2012), Mexico: the first steps toward Basic Income. In R. Caputo (ed.), *Basic Income Guarantee and Politics: International Experiences and Perspectives on the Viability of Income Guarantee*, New York, NY: Palgrave Macmillan, pp. 217–33.

# INDEX

*New Perspectives on Health, Disability, Welfare and the Labour Market*, First Edition.
Edited by Colin Lindsay, Bent Greve, Ignazio Cabras, Nick Ellison and Stephen Kellett.
© 2015 John Wiley & Sons, Ltd. Published 2015 by John Wiley & Sons, Ltd.